Natural Remedies for Women

By Charles Silverman N.D.

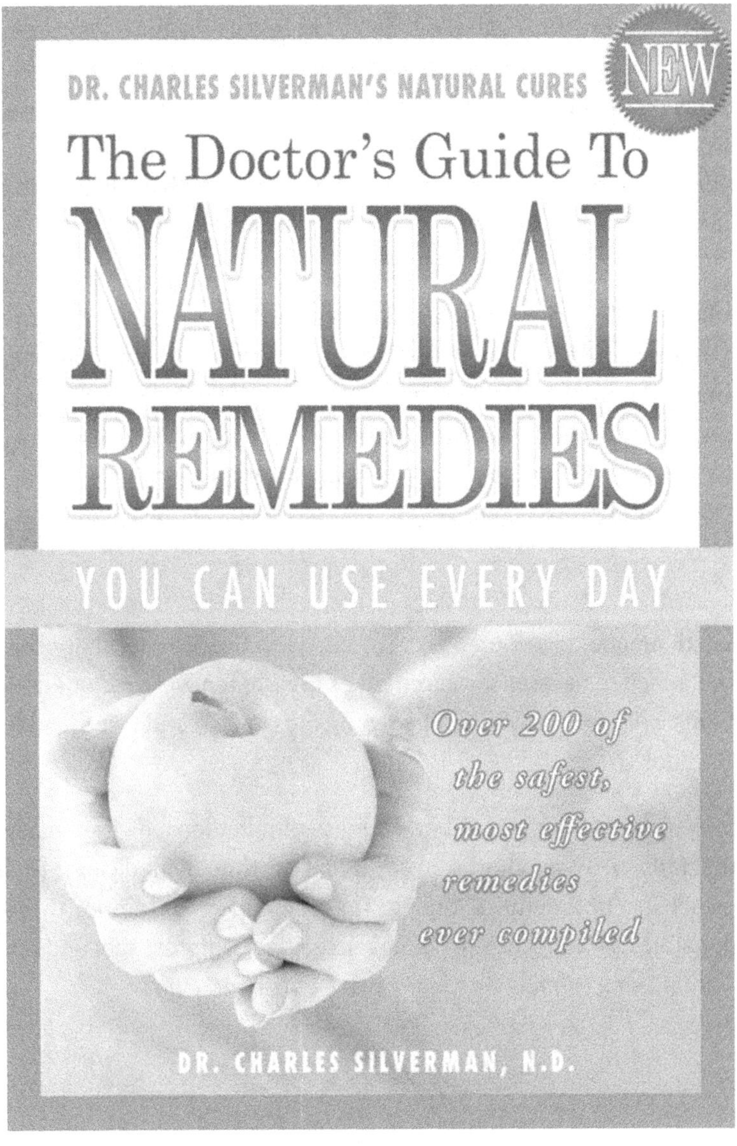

DR. CHARLES SILVERMAN'S NATURAL CURES · NEW

The Doctor's Guide To

NATURAL REMEDIES

YOU CAN USE EVERY DAY

Over 200 of the safest, most effective remedies ever compiled

DR. CHARLES SILVERMAN, N.D.

When it comes to health women are hunted by completely different array of diseases than men. Although they might look similar in appearance men and women´s bodies cannot be compare. Women have a long list of health conditions that need a very specific approach, for instance menopause a condition that tortures women in their later years, or vaginal and urinary infections are common complaints, none of these health problems affect men.

Many illnesses do affect women and men alike, however, the symptoms associated with them can be very different and so is the treatment approach. Some natural remedies used for treating a common cold in men could actually have an undesirable effect in women. With these ideas as a backbone I came to the conclusion that women need their own natural healing encyclopedia, and that is how this book came to be.

This health manual for women was created with the premise that only the most safe and effective natural home remedies for women were included. Hundreds of patients were interviewed and only the most successful treatments made it into this book.

For twenty years I have prescribed various combinations of vitamins, minerals, essential fatty acids, and herbs, in addition to orthodox medicines, to help women achieve optimum well-being. The tremendous difference these nutritional supplements can make never ceases to impress me, and I firmly believe that using them is worth any extra effort and expense.

Many women prefer the process of healing to be a natural one, the good news is that there are naturopathic means of treating many of the discomforts caused by illnesses.

I will not take time and precious paper "real estate" going on and on about things that are obvious to you, instead we are going to jump head first into each illness and health problem for women. So select and use any of the remedies you will find in this book with peace of main, knowing that only the best remedies, researched by professionals are at your disposal at any time.

ABOUT

Charles Silverman N.D., a Naturalist and Herbalist since 1979, is the author of the Home Made Medicine e-book and the www.HomeMadeMedicine.com Web site. Charles lives in Miami, FL and has dedicated a major part of his life to the preparation of natural remedies and natural products to help people with allergies and chemical intolerance. He has traveled around the world from Canada, Germany, France, and India to the mountains of Peru and Argentina (South America) researching and studying the different domestic species of herbs and plants. His articles are published on several web sites like ezinearticles.com and naturalhealthweb.com and he is regularly interviewed by various publications and newspapers like the Montgomery News of Alabama.

All his knowledge has been transferred to his web site and now to this amazing book, that takes advantage of the latest technology in order to bring you the most complete guide for home healing ever made.

Migraine:

Migraine is the term used to describe a severe pain in the head. This can be caused by the contraction or dilatation of blood vessels in the brain and the irregular nerve activity mainly in the meninges.
Migraine is caused by the stimulation of the trigeminal nerve which release a substance inducing inflammation and also sends messages to pain receptors in the meninges.

People who suffer from migraines often are between the ages of 20 and 30. However, children can have migraines too but their symptoms are shown as colic, periodic abdominal pains, vomiting, dizziness and severe motion sickness. Then these symptoms will disappear, focusing in the exact problem, painful headaches. Almost every person who suffers from migraines will have some symptoms before having one.

There are five phases

5

1. The day before the person has a migraine there may be a very noticeable change in the mood or problems remembering things or an alteration in one or all of the five senses or he/she could have speech problems.

2. A moment before the migraine begins some people see flashes or experience numbness of the hands and mouth.

3. Once the migraine starts the pain could be overwhelming. It may be at one or both sides of the head. You can experience some nausea along with sensitivity in the neck and scalp.

4. The headaches will soon disappear including the nausea.

5. After these symptoms you may feel tired, without energy and will want to sleep.

A migraine can be due to allergies, constipation, stress, liver malfunction, too much or too little sleep, emotional changes, hormonal changes, suns glare, flashing lights, poor exercise, dental problems, low blood sugar and changes in the barometric pressure.

We recommend:

• Eat a diet that is low in carbohydrates and high in protein. Try to include in your diet almonds, watercress, parsley, fennel, garlic, cherries and pineapple.

• Avoid alcohol, processed meat (hot dogs), chocolates, aspirin, avocados, beer, bananas, canned fish, cabbage, eggplant, dairy products, potatoes, hard cheeses, tomatoes, wine, red plums, yeast, raspberries, salt, meat, cereal, grains, bread, fried foods and greasy foods.

• Do not miss any meal. Instead eat small, nutritious meals and have some snacks if needed.

• Take only hypoallergenic supplements.

• Get plenty of exercise.

• During the day massage your neck and the back of your head several times to relieve tension.

• Try to be always in a calm ambient, avoid strong odors and high altitudes.

• Do not smoke and do not allow people to smoke in front of you.

• Take a cup of strong coffee to relieve pain caused by migraine.

• To prevent or control the migraine supplements are needed such as:

Calcium + Magnesium. They help to regulate muscle tone and to transmit nerve impulses throughout the body and to the brain.

• Primrose oil has an anti-inflammatory agent that keeps the blood vessels from constricting.

- Multivitamin and mineral formulas are necessary daily to complement the nutrients we do not include in our diet.

- Rutin removes toxic metals which may cause migraines.

- Garlic is a potent detoxifier.

- Vitamin C with bioflavonoids helps in producing an anti-stress adrenal hormone and enhances immunity.

- In addition are a variety of herbs that can help control and relieve migraines:

Cordyceps reduces anxiety and stress and at the same time promotes sleep.

Feverfew reduces discomfort and pain. Caution: Avoid during pregnancy.

- Gingko Biloba extract enhances cerebral circulation.

• Iris versicolor relieves pain and discomfort.

• To alleviate migraines massage one drop of peppermint oil into each temple.

• You can also drink one cup infusion of Hops or take ½ tsp. extract 3 times daily.

• At the first sign of a migraine take Black Willow, Jamaican Dogwood, Passion Flower, Valerian or Wood Betony to ease the pain.

• To ease pain, instead of taking pain killers that have serious side effects, try making these teas, are natural and have no side effects.

1 tsp. Feverfew leaves.

1 tsp. Peppermint leaves.

1 cup boiling water.

Mix all the herbs in a nonmetallic container and cover with the boiling water, steep for 30minutes, then strain. If you want, add honey for taste. Take one tbs. at a time. Throughout the day you should drink more than one cup of the tea.

Endometriosis

Endometriosis occurs when tissue from the lining of the uterus (the endometrium) attaches itself elsewhere in the abdomen. This brings a wide array of problems especially before menstruation when the lining expands.

Endometriosis affects about 10% of women in the U.S. However European females rarely get this disease. It is very painful, cramps in the abdomen are quite common. Other symptoms are, intestinal gas, excessive menstrual bleeding, insomnia and depression. This disease can cause infertility.

The reason for this disorder is not clear but what we know is that excessive amount of estrogen has an impact on the severity of endometriosis.

The drugs usually prescribed for the disease causes vaginal dryness, low sex drive, and menopause symptoms. Herbs can offer some help without complications.

We recommend

• Burdock is one of the best herbs to clean the liver and as we know estrogen is excreted by the liver. An efficient liver will rid estrogen more quickly.

• To reduce bleeding, inflammation and cramps, use wild yam, primrose, and ginger. Since these symptoms are similar to the ones for PMS, use the remedies we suggest in the PMS section of this book.

Endometriosis Tea.

1 tsp. vitex berries.

1 tsp. echinacea root.

1 tsp. wild yam rhizome.

1 tsp. cramp bark.

½ tsp. horsetail stalks.

½ tsp. red raspberry.

½ tsp. motherwort.

1 quart water.

Mix herbs and water in a saucepan and boil. Simmer for 5 minutes and steep for another 10 minutes. Strain and drink 2 cups a day.

The herb vitex berry controls estrogen which is one of the causes of endometriosis. By controlling levels of estrogen, this herb helps reduce the symptoms.

To reduce the size of the uterus use raspberry extract. It has been used to reduce bleeding for hundreds of years.

Infertility

Infertility is usually referred to as the incapacity to conceive after a year or more of regular sexual activity during the time of ovulation. Infertility affects 6 million couples in the United States and finding the reason for infertility can be difficult. There are many conditions that can cause infertility, some of them require surgery to be corrected others are caused by hormonal imbalance. Herbs can help in almost all cases in which hormones are the reason for infertility. That's why you should first find out the cause of the infertility before choosing a specific herbal treatment.

Some of the causes of infertility are:

• Stress can prevent ovulation.

• Very athletic women, with very low body fat, stop ovulating. This is a common problem for professional athletes.

TIP: Did you know that some women develop antibodies to their partners' sperm, in effect becoming allergic to them?

• Some contraceptives disrupted the hormonal balance causing infertility.

• Women with depress immune systems often are unable to become pregnant or they usually miscarry early in the pregnancy.

• Irregular menstrual cycles can make it very hard for some women to become pregnant.

•Endometriosis causes infertility. See endometriosis .

We recommend

• A study done in United States showed that women suffering from stress were able to become pregnant after learning relaxation techniques. See stress in this e-book.

• Studies on don quai show that it helps ovaries function better and

15

it restores normal cycles.

• The herb vitex has been researched in Germany. That research has shown that vitex increases the levels of three hormones: progesterone, prolactin and luteinizing hormone (LH). These hormones help women become pregnant, sustain pregnancy and produce milk.

• Wild yam helps the uterus during pregnancy thus reducing the chances of miscarriage.

Fertility Herbal Treatment.

1 tsp. don quai root.

1 tsp. siberian ginseng root.

1 tsp. vitex berries.

1 tsp. motherwort leaves.

1 tsp. cramp bark.

1 tsp. wild yam rhizome.

1 quart water.

Mix herbs and simmer for 10 minutes. Steep for 10 minutes, strain and drink 2 cups a day.

• If you are not allergic to bee pollen, include it in your diet. Royal jelly is very helpful as well.

TIP: Did you know that alcohol prevents implantation of the fertilized egg in women?

Irregular Menstruation and hormonal Tonic.

1 tsp. vitex berries.

1 tsp. don quai root.

1 tsp. licorice root.

½ tsp. motherwort leaves.

½ tsp. siberian ginseng root.

1 quart of water.

Mix all ingredients, simmer for 10 minutes and steep for 20 minutes. Strain and drink 1 cup a day during menstruation until ovulation. If you are not menstruating, drink throughout the month.

TIP: Did you know that Ulcer medications cimetidine (Tagamet) and ranitidine (Zantac) may decrease the sperm count in some men and even produce impotence?

Miscarriage Prevention.

1 tsp. false unicorn root.

1 tsp. cramp bark.

½ tsp. red raspberry leaves.

½ tsp. wild yam root.

3 cups water.

Boil water and herbs and simmer for 10 minutes. Steep for 10 minutes, strain and drink 8 cups during the course of a day. If you find this to be too much liquid, you can use these herbs in a tincture and take 2 drops each false unicorn and cramp bark, 1 drop each red raspberry and wild yam 4 times a day.

Vaginal Infections.

Douche for vaginal infections.

3 drops lavender essential oil.

3 tea tree essential oil.

3 cups of warm water.

3 tbs.. of yogurt.

Mix ingredients in a douche bag. Use as needed for a week.

Vaginal infection tea.

1 tsp. cramp bark.

1 tsp. burdock root.

1 tsp. echinacea root.

1 tsp. oregon grape root.

1 tsp. vitex seeds.

1 quart of water.

Mix all herbs and simmer for 10 minutes, remove from heat and steep for 15 minutes. Strain and drink 3 cups a day.

• Barberry has remarkable infection fighting properties.

• Goldenseal used as an external topic or vaginal suppository is very helpful for all types of infections.

• Colloidal silver is a natural antibiotic that kills many types of bacteria.

• Tea tree oil is good for vaginitis. A cream made with tea tree oil is very effective against fungal infections, herpes blisters, wartsand other types of infections. A tea tree oil suppository has been used for years to fight yeast infections.

TIP: Did you know that eating yogurt and applying yogurt directly to the vagina, helps fight infections and relieves inflammation?

• Peel and blend 4 pieces of garlic and 1 cup of apple cider vinegar and 2 cups of warm water. Strain and wash vagina with the liquid.

Fibrocystic breast:

Fibrocystic breast is a condition that develops when fluid is not being evacuated fast enough from the breast causing cysts to form in them. These lumps move around the breast, grow and shrink, but they are benign.

Normally the fluids in the breast are transported out by the lymphatic system. But if there is too much fluid some may get deposited in different areas of the breast. Tissue grows around them creating these lumps. Like we said before these cysts are harmless but they should be monitored and a woman should check her breasts frequently in order to find and control the cysts. Frequent mammograms are recommended too.

Discomfort, tenderness, and noticeable growth are normal especially around menstrual periods when estrogen levels change. The cysts may disappear after the monthly period. However if the lump is hard and does not move freely and does not go away, check with a doctor immediately.

We recommend

TIP: Did you know that the herb Saw Palmetto helps increase breast size especially at puberty?

• Coenzyme Q10 is very important to remove toxins from the body and help control fibrocystic breasts.

• In many studies Primrose oil has been shown to reduce size of lumps.

• Take vitamin E. It's an antioxidant that protects breast tissue against fibrocystic breasts.

• Vitamin B6 manages fluids and hormone levels.

- The herb astragalus increases circulation to the surface of the skin helping to evacuate toxins.

- Black cohosh regulates menstrual periods and hormone levels reducing the chance of developing fibrocystic breasts.

- Castor oil is used frequently to shrink the size of cysts if used during several months.

- Burdock is very helpful in draining fluid and removing toxins reducing fibrocystic breasts.

- Poke root cleans the lymphatic fluid and clears abscesses present in fibrocystic breasts.

- Chasteberry balances estrogen helping reduce the development of cysts if used for several months.

- Examine your breast once a month. This can help detect early tumors or fibrocystic breasts.

• Don't drink coffee, regular tea, colas or chocolate and any foods that contain caffeine as it has been proven to increase fibrocystic breasts.

Breast Cyst tea.

1 tsp. burdock root.

1 tsp. mullein leaves.

1 tsp. dandelion root.

1/2 tsp. prickly ash bark.

1/2 tsp. cleavers leaves.

1 quart water.

Mix ingredients and drink 2 cups a day.

Breast compress.

1/2 tsp. calendula flowers tincture.

10 drops lavender essential oil.

3 drops ginger essential oil.

3 drops chamomile essential oil.

1 cup warm water.

1 cotton cloth.

Mix all ingredients, soak rag in the solution and place it over the area where the cysts are for 5 minutes, then repeat.

Frigidity:

Frigidity is mostly used to describe a sexual dysfunction in women and is the inability to experience pleasure from sexual intercourse. It is characterized by a lack of sexual desire and responsiveness due to traumatic sexual experience or other unpleasant episodes during childhood or as an adolescent. It is caused by psychological origin, stemming from fear, anxiety, guilt, depression, problems with the partner and/or feelings of inferiority.

Some women find intercourse painful due to poor lubrication, inadequate stimulation, some illness or infection or it can be related to other physical causes. The pain that these women experience causes them to shrink and fear from sexual contact with the partner. Vitamin deficiency can cause a deficiency in estrogen levels and lead to improper lubrication. Low sexual desire can also be due to a chronic illness, the use of some medications, low testosterone levels or a certain medical condition.

We recommend:

• Make sure that in your diet you are including a good quantity of alfalfa sprouts, avocados, eggs that come fresh from hens (avoid the ones stored cold in the supermarket), olive oil, pumpkin seeds, other seeds and nuts, soy and sesame oil and wheat.

• Avoid red meat, poultry and products containing sugar.

• Avoid smoggy conditions. Smog is highly toxic and dangerous and affects the entire immune function and hormonal activity in the body.

• Also herbs can help cope with the problem. Here are the most common:

Chives contain minerals required for the creation of sex hormones.

Damiana the " woman's sexuality herb", is the most popular aphrodisiac plant. This plant contains alkaloids that stimulate the nerves and organs. It's perfect for supporting the sexual organs and enhancing sexual pleasure.

Kava kava helps deal with anxiety and nervousness. Caution: Not recommended for pregnant women or nursing mothers. It should not be taken together with alcohol, barbiturates, antidepressants, antipsycotic drugs or any other substance that acts upon the central nervous system.

Wild yam contains a natural steroid that gives vigor to lovemaking and rejuvenates.

There are other great herbs used in promoting energy and sexuality such as: fo-ti, gotu kola, sarsaparrilla and saw palmetto.

• Some supplements can help such as:

Kelp: 2,000-2,500 mg daily; it's a good source of iodine and other important minerals.

Vitamin B complex: 100 mg of each major B vitamin twice daily; aids in reducing anxiety and calms the nervous system.

Vitamin E: Start taking 200-400 IU daily and increase slowly to 1,600

IU daily; it's necessary for the good functioning of the reproductive system and glands. Use the d-alphatocopherol form.

TIP: Did you know that the herb Saw Palmetto helps increase breast size especially at puberty.

P.M.S. (Prementrual Syndrome):

Prementrual syndrome is the most common gynecological complaint of women and it affects about 60% of them. The symptoms appear one or two weeks before menstruation starts, and they include: abdominal bloating and cramps, acne, anxiety, breast tenderness and swelling and mood changes.

During menstruation there is an imbalance in hormones and brain activity and it is believed that too much estrogen, uneven levels of progesterone and an inability to cope with hormone changes are the main causes of PMS. But the real reason as to why this condition affects so many women is unknown.

About 5% of women suffer such severe complications that they are incapable of functioning normally during this period. Others claim symptoms interfere with their daily activities.

Using herbs we can return hormone levels to their normal level and proper diet can help reduce many of the symptoms. The final result is a body that is back in balance without using drugs and without experiencing any side effects.

We recommend

• Take magnesium 1,000 mg. a day. Deficiencies have been linked to PMS.

• Take calcium 1,500 mg. a day to help reduce some symptoms.

• Take Vitamin B6 to reduce water retention and increase blood circulation to the female organs.

• Take Vitamin E to help reduce breast soreness.

TIP: Did you know that caffeine makes the changes of suffering from severe PMS symptoms 4 times greater?

• Black cohosh relieves premenstrual tension, menstrual cramps and water retention and helps control mood changes.
• Dandelion root is a very powerful diuretic that helps evacuate

excess water and bloating but is safer then commercial diuretics because it does not deplete potassium. Another important quality is that it helps the liver discard estrogen thus relieving PMS.

• Dong Quai reduces cramps, pain and mood changes and regulates phytoestrogen leveling the hormones.

• Maca regulates hormones according to the body's need. It reduces acne occurrences and contains minerals and vitamins needed during PMS.

• Wild yam regulates levels of estrogen and progesterone. It relaxes the muscles and nerves.

• Studies have shown that Chaste tree regulates hormonal changes, reduces anxiety, mood changes and water retention and breast pain.

Mix the following ingredients:
1 tsp. of black cohosh root.
1 tsp. of passionflower.
1 tsp. of oregon grape root.

1 tsp. white willow bark.

2 cup of water.

Boil for 30 minutes, strain, take one tbsp. per hour.

Make a tea mixing:

1 tsp. black haw.

1 tsp. licorice root.

1 tsp. evening primrose.

1 tsp. milk thistle.

4 cups of boiling water.

Let it steep for 30 minutes, strain, drink 2 cups a day.

Mix the following ingredients

1 tsp. vitex berries.

1 tsp. wild yam rhizome.

½ tsp. burdock root.

½ tsp. dandelion root.

4 cups of boiling water.

Steep for 30 minutes, strain and drink 1 or 2 cups a day.

• Jamaican dogwood is a strong pain reliever, sedative and antispasmodic. Very helpful for muscular back pain, asthma, menstrual pain, insomnia, toothaches and nervous conditions.

Relaxing PMS Remedy.

1 tsp. Valerian rhizome tincture.

½ tsp. catnip leaves tincture.

½ tsp. passionflower leaves tincture.

1/4 tsp. peppermint leaves tincture.

Mix all ingredients and take a dropperful 4 times a day.

Menstrual cramp oil.

2 ounces Saint John's Wart oil.

8 drops Lavander essential oil.

8 drops Marjoram essential oil.

8 drops Chamomile essential oil.

Mix all ingredients and rub the lower obdomen with it as needed. This formula can be used for back pain or any muscle related cramp.

Menstrual bleeding control tincture.

1 tsp. shepherd's purse leaf tincture.

1 tsp. yarrow leaf tincture.

1/2 tsp. red raspberry leaf tincture.

1/2 tsp. vitex berry tincture.

Mix all ingredients and take 1/2 a dropperful 4 times a day.

Stretch Marks:

It is very common that almost every woman at a specific time in her life will develop stretch marks. Others simply have a generic predisposition to stretch marks and get them everywhere while still others never develop stretch marks at all.

They look like reddish lines across the body, and with time, they will turn white. In pregnancy it is common to have them due to the fact that the skin is stretching very rapidly to accommodate the baby and the milk stored in the breasts.

Once the stretch marks develop they will stay with you forever; however, with time they will be less noticeable. The only way to avoid stretch marks is to prevent them.

We recommend:

• It is very important to exercise in order to get rid of stretch marks; toning your muscles helps your skin firm thus preventing stretch marks.

• Make sure that in your diet you are getting plenty of protein and foods rich in Vitamin C and Vitamin E which promote good tissue growth.

• Massaging your body with olive oil or Vitamin E may help.

• You can also try this homemade recipe: Mix one ounce of carrier oil (try avocado, sweet almond, jojoba, they are the best) with seven drops of lavender and five drops of chamomile. Massage into the body.

• Apply cocoa butter and/ or elastin cream thoughout the body as directed on the label. These are very good for stretch marks.

Here is another good recipe:

½ cup virgin olive oil.

1/4 cup aloe vera gel.

liquid from 6 capsules of Vitamin E.

liquid from 4 capsules of Vitamin A.

Mix all the ingredients together in a blender. Then pour the mixture into a jar and store it in the fridge. Apply the oil externally all over the places where the stretch marks commonly appear (abdomen, hips, thighs and breasts). If you do this consistently every day, you may prevent stretch marks.

Varicose Veins:

Varicose veins are abnormally enlarged veins that appear close to the skin's surface. They occur usually in the calves and thighs and are the result of malfunctioning valves inside the veins often caused by prolonged pressure or obstruction of the veins.

Varicose veins can develop in people from standing or sitting for long periods of time, poor exercise, pregnancy, excessive weight, prolonged constipation, and habitually sitting with legs crossed. Also, heavy lifting puts increased pressure on legs increasing the likelihood of developing varicose veins. Heart failure, liver disease and abdominal tumors can contribute to the formation of varicose veins. Heredity is also a factor for many individuals. A deficiency of Vitamin C and bioflavonoids can weaken the collagen structure in the vein walls which can lead to varicose veins.

Varicose veins are very common and affect approximately 10% of the population. More women than men are affected. In some cases if varicose veins are not treated properly, some complications can emerge. The most common characteristics are: swelling, restlessness, leg sores, itching, leg cramps, feeling of heaviness in the legs and fatigue.

We recommend:

• Eat a balanced diet that includes plenty of fish, fresh fruits and vegetables. The diet also has to be low in fat and carbohydrates.

• Eat as many blackberries and cherries as you can. They help prevent varicose veins and if you have them they may ease the symptoms.

• Including ginger, onions, garlic and pineapple in your diet is beneficial.

• Your diet has to be high in fiber to prevent constipation and keep the bowels clean.

• Avoid as much as possible sugar, ice cream, fried foods, peanuts, junk foods, cheeses, tobacco, salt, alcohol, animal protein, and processed and refined foods.

• Do a daily routine of exercise. Walking, swimming and bicycling all promote good circulation. It is very important to maintain a healthy weight.

• Do not wear tight clothes because they restrict blood flow.

• At least once a day, elevate your legs above the heart level for 20 minutes to alleviate symptoms.

• Avoid standing or sitting for long periods of time, crossing your legs, doing heavy lifting and putting any unnecessary pressure on your legs.

• If you sit at a desk all day, make sure you take breaks to walk around. You can also flex your muscles and wiggle your toes to increase blood flow. If it is possible, try to rest your feet on an object that is elevated from the floor when seated.

• If you have to stand for long periods of time, shift your weight between your feet, stand on your toes, or take breaks and walk around to alleviate pressure.

• Elevate your feet, as much as possible, at home while watching TV or sitting down to read.

• To ease pain and stimulate circulation, fill a tub with cold water and simulate walking.

• Avoid scratching the itchy skin above varicose veins. This can cause ulceration and bleeding.

• After bathing, apply Castor oil over the varicose veins affected and massage into your legs from the feet up.

• Also herbs can play a key role in treating varicose veins. Here are some helpful herbs:

• Aloe vera gel is a cooling and soothing treatment for varicose veins.

• Bilberry supports the health of connective tissue.

• Bromelain can help reduce the risk of clot formation in the blood vessels.

• To improve the circulation in the legs, Butchers broom, ginkgo biloba, gotu kola and hawthorn berries are very good.

• To relieve pain and inflammation use Cayenne. It also expands blood vessels, reducing stress on the capillaries.

• To alleviate tissue swelling use Dandelion. Dandelion reduces water retention.

• To stimulate blood flow, bathe the affected areas in white oak bark herb tea 3 times daily or simmer, but do not boil, a strong tea and use it to make compresses. Apply to the painful areas.

Here are some home recipes that might help:

2 tsp black cohosh root.

4 tsp Ginkgo biloba leaves.

2 cups boiling water.

Combine the herbs. Pour the boiling water over the herb mixture; soak for 30 minutes, strain. Take 2 to 3 tbsp at a time, repeat up to 6 times daily to improve circulation.

Topical formula.

1 tsp ocotilo bark.

1 tsp yarrow.

1 tsp witch hazel bark.

2 cups of water.

Combine all ingredients in a pan and cover, boil until reduced to one cup; cool and strain. Apply topically to reduce discomfort. Use as needed.

Vein Reducer.

½ tsp horse chestnut powder.

2 cups water.

Mix and moisten a sterile cotton gauze cloth with the mixture. Rub gently over the affected area. This is to reduce discomfort over inflamed veins.

Wrinkles:

Wrinkles form when the skin thins and loses its elasticity. The appearance of some wrinkles is due to aging and is the most common skin problem for women. One of the first signs of wrinkles normally appear around the eye and is called " crow's feet." As time goes by the cheeks and lips are the next thing we notice. As we age, our skin becomes thinner and dryer, both factors contribute to the formation of wrinkles.

There are many factors that can contribute in the development of wrinkles some of which are: diet and nutrition, muscle tone, pollution, habitual facial expressions, chemicals, stress, improper skin care, and lifestyle habits such as smoking.

The most important factor is sun exposure which is your skin's worst enemy because it dries the skin and leads to the generation of free radicals that can damage skin cells. Research shows that 90% of what we think are signs of age are actually signs of over exposure to sunlight. Furthermore, approximately 70% of sun damage comes from everyday activities such as driving and walking to and from your car.

The ultraviolet-A rays that cause this enormous damage are present all day long in all seasons. These ultraviolet-A rays wear away the elasticity of the skin, causing wrinkling. The worst part is that the effects of the sun are cumulative, although they may not be noticeable for many years.

TIP:Did you know that natural beauty products are not always as advertised?

Manufacturers say that their products contain natural ingredients but the reality is that they contain tiny amounts compared to the artificial substances used. You find out by looking at the label of the product. The ingredients are listed in descending order, starting with the greatest amount contained. For example, a product may be labeled as rosemary, but the label shows only chemicals and artificial substances and not a drop of pure rosemary.

We recommend:

• Eat a balanced diet including fruits, vegetables, whole grain foods, seeds, nuts and legumes.

• Drink plenty of fluids every day. This help to keep the skin hydrated and flush away toxins.

• Obtain fatty acids from cold pressed vegetable oils.

• Avoid alcohol, caffeine and cigarettes. They dry the skin and encourage the development of wrinkles. Also the smoking habit uses the lips' muscles hundreds of times a day which contributes to wrinkling.

• Always protect your skin from the sun by applying a sunscreen with a sun protection factor (SPF) of at least 15 to all exposed areas of the skin.

• Avoid alcohol-based products. Use hazel or an herbal, floral water instead.

• Avoid using harsh soaps or solid cleansing creams. Use natural oils such as avocado oil to remove dirt and makeup.

• Do not apply heavy oils around the eye area before going to bed. Because it might cause the eye to be puffy in the morning.

• Take Vitamin E to protect against free radicals that can damage the skin and contribute to aging and wrinkles.

• Take Vitamin C to promote the formation of collagen, a protein that gives the skin flexibility. It also fights free radicals and strengthens the capillaries that feed the skin.

• Take Silica. It is important for skin strength and elasticity and also, stimulates collagen formation.

• Take Vitamin A. It is necessary for healing and the construction of new skin tissue.

• Take Vitamin B complex + Vitamin B12. They are anti stress and anti-aging vitamins.

• Take primrose or black currant seed oil. They are good healers for dermatitis, acne and others skin disorders.

• Use a collagen cream because it is very good for dry skin.

• Use elastin cream to help smooth existing wrinkles and prevent the appearance of new ones.

• To alleviate puffy eyes, peel a cucumber, cool it and place it in the eye area for 10 minutes. Repeat if necessary.

• To cleanse the pores, rub mush tomatoes over your face, then rinse.

• To protect your skin from free radical damage, add a few drops of green tea extract to your lotions or astringents.

• To moisture your skin, mash together grapes and honey, enough to make a paste, apply over your face as a mask. Leave it for 30 minutes then rinse away.

• To remove dead cells and improve skin texture, rub a small handful of dry short grain rice against your face for a couple of minutes.

• To soften and nourish the skin, mash half an avocado and apply over the face. Leave it on until it dries, then rinse with warm water. Your pregnancy and your baby:

Pregnancy the most special time for you, your partner and your baby, who in just 40 weeks will be coming into your life for ever. This is a time to be treated with great respect and awe. This is a time to do the best for you and your baby.

For your baby, this time of peace and security will depend upon our lifestyle and the lifestyles of those around you.

Tip: Studies have shown that women who are more fit tend to have shorter, easier labor.

What you eat and drink will construct your baby's body. Also mother nature ensures that it will do the very best that can be done in the physical developments of you and your child but much of the responsibility lies on the parent's shoulders. Special care can and should be taken and herbs can play a key role in this important time of your life.

Nature offers an abundance of plants and herbs for all the stages of your birthing process. Some plants or herbs may be used at specific times and others throughout your pregnancy, to ease, aid and tone the tissue and to facilitate the birth itself.

We all know that synthetic drugs are to be avoided during pregnancy. That's why a natural approach to healing should be considered throughout the time the baby's in the mother's womb. Natural techniques can help you increase your energy, consolidate emotional serenity and also help you deal with the comforts and problems that may emerge as you proceed through your pregnancy and prepare for the birth of your baby. This involves a good diet, regular exercise and plenty of rest.

During your pregnancy is the right time to consider the practice of other techniques such as massage sessions, herbalism, homeopathy, acupressure, visualization, and other mind/body techniques that can make your pregnancy easier and more comfortable for you and for your baby as well.

In this part of the book we'll offer precise amounts of herbs, homeopathic remedies and aroma therapy oils that will help you find a cure for some problem that might emerge or to just relax during this beautiful experience, as well as suggested dietary or vitamin/mineral supplementation.

Back Pain:

About 80% of adults suffer from back pain at some time in their lives. Backaches are categorized as acute and chronic. Acute pain is caused by movement or excessive use of the back which can injure the muscles, ligaments, bones, tendons.

Chronic pain is a recurring backache that restricts of normal movements for no particular reason and can also affect the tendons, ligaments and bones.

Problems with some organs can cause back pain as well, for example, kidney infection, prostate problems, female pelvic disorder, bladder and even constipation can be felt in the lower back.

Back pain is very common during pregnancy due to the considerable anatomical changes and stress in the body. Carrying a child changes the position of your internal organs putting a huge amount of pressure on the lower spine. The increase in body weight, the muscle relaxing effects of the hormone progesterone and the change in your center of gravity contribute to the problem. That's why every day as your baby grows it's harder to get up and down from chairs and beds.

If you have back pain you can also feel muscle aches, locked areas in your back, stiff neck and your whole body will ache.

Other causes of back pain can be poor postural habits, strains, microtrauma, muscle tension and nutritional deficiencies. When repeated episodes of injury are added to this mix, the discs become thin, deteriorated or ruptured. These events can also lead to arthritic related conditions. With nerves close by, swelling or compression in the spine often results in neuritis, lumbar neuralgia, or sciatica.

Herbal medicines are used in these conditions with far more safety then drugs especially in pregnant women.

We recommend
•Ask someone to massage the affected area with herbal oils using knuckles and increasing pressure slowly. After a few minutes you will feel less discomfort. This gets rid of tension and relaxes the muscles in that area.

•Every time you lift something, remember to bend your knees first. This will prevent your lower back from getting tense and causing damage to your spine and back muscles.

•Never twist while lifting as this can have a bad effect on your vertebrates.

•Avoid lifting heavy objects in the last couple of weeks of your pregnancy.

•Do not sit in couches. Always sit in firm chairs supporting the lumbar area with a pillow. This will help you keep your waist and lower back in the proper position.

•Apply St. john's Wort directly to the back area. CAUTION: Do not suntan as this oil makes your skin very sensitive to the sun.

•Do not wear high heel shoes. They change your center of gravity even more, increasing the risk of falling and they put more pressure on your back. Instead wear well fitted, well-padded flat shoes that support your feet and provide ample room for your toes.

•Try to sleep with pillows supporting your back, legs and belly.

•Here are some homeopathic remedies that will help you with back pains, Cimicifuga, Kali carbonica. Lincopodium, Nux vomica and Arnica.

•Black Haw contains compounds very similar to the ones found in aspirin. It relieves spasms and neuralgia of back and neck, sciatica, leg cramps, tension headaches and wry neck.

•Boswellia is a strong anti-inflammatory which reduces stiffness and pain. It has to be used for at least 4 weeks in chronic cases. It improves circulation around ligaments, joints and tendons.

•Jamaican dogwood is a strong pain reliever, sedative and antispasmodic. It's very helpful for muscular back pain, asthma, menstrual pain, insomnia, toothaches, and nervous conditions.

•Dong quai has 1.5 times the analgesic activity of aspirin. It relieves back pain, cramping, muscular spasms and inflammation.

•The herb Cat's claw grows in South America has been researched and proven to reduce inflammation while boosting the immune system. The studies also discovered that cat's claw contains anti arthritic compounds and is currently being used to treat people with rheumatoid arthritis.

•Take Vitamin E to protect and improve joint mobility.

•Bromelain comes from the stem of the pineapple. It contains anti-inflammatory blocks, reduces swelling, pain and damage to joints. A study done on 200 people showed a 75% greater reduction in inflammation than the ones obtained using drugs. Finally in the last few years bromelain is being used in hospitals across U.S.

•Wild yam, is used for back pain characterized by sharp, knifelike sensations.

•Barberry is used for low back pain often related to kidney weakness. Good also for sciatica and neuralgia with radiating pain.

•Horsetail has high amounts of silica which is essential for bones and connective tissue.

•Eat alfalfa or take alfalfa extract in capsules. It contains all the necessary nutrients to alleviate back pain.

TIP: A homemade ice pack can be made by mixing 2 parts water and 1 part alcohol in a nylon bag and freezing it. The bag will be flexible thus molding to the body and it will not sweat.

•When pain hits suddenly, drink two large glasses of pure water. Dehydration can cause back pain.

•Several studies done in Scandinavia on smoking and non smoking twins have shown that smoking greatly aggravates problems in the disks. It's always advisable to quit smoking.

•Rhus toxicodendrom is a homeopathic remedy that relieves stiffness.

Breast-feeding:

Breast-feeding is the act of naturally feeding an infant with milk produced in the mother's breast. This has great deal of benefits for the baby. Not only is breast milk healthier but the action of feeding the child is a moment of love in which the baby learns to bond, smell, and caress with his or her mother as she gives nourishment and affection.

Without a doubt breast milk is the best food for a newborn, nothing comes closer to providing all the nutrients that the baby will need later in life. Breast milk is much easier to digest then any formula on the market, and at the same time it provides protection against infections, prevents future food allergies, helps the growth of healthy teeth, and most important it improves brain development. Studies have shown that breast-fed babies are more intelligent than formula fed babies.

However, many mothers stop breast-feeding after the third or fourth month switching to formula and later to cows' milk. This certainly robs the baby of the special qualities that breast milk offers. Infants that stop nursing before the fourth month are at risk of developing asthma, food and respiratory allergies, intestinal bacteria, and oral weaknesses (poor tooth development).

Sometimes a mother cannot breast-fed her baby due to a number of reasons, such as, low quality of milk, breast pain, infection, etc. That's when herbs come into play, many midwives have used them for years to improve quality and quantity of milk, to fight infection and much more. Take a look at the following conditions and the natural ways to treat them.

Low quality or quantity of milk

Low quality of milk can be caused by medications or a poor diet. Many antibiotics contaminate the milk and a diet high in caffeine may cause colic and sleeping problems. For the baby, it's very important that the mother keeps eating a well balance diet after giving birth, and preferably foods with no traces of pesticides. These poisons become highly concentrated in the milk.

The use of a breast pump may inhibit the production of milk, lowering the amount available to the baby, this gives the false idea that the infant should be changed to formula in order for it to be satisfied when, in fact, the problem is the quantity of milk that the mother is producing.

Herbs can help with both of these common problems.

We recommend

• Eat alfalfa or take it in capsules, it stimulates lactation, improves quality and quantity of milk.

• Chaste tree increases flow of milk by affecting pituitary's prolactin secretion.

• Chinese use a herb called codonopsis to increase lactation and strengthen the blood.

• Goat's rue is an herb that has been used by midwives for hundreds of years to improve breast milk production by as much as 50%.

• Vervain encourages milk secretion and flow. It also increases absorption of nutrients from food and helps with postpartum depression.

• Milk thistle promotes production of milk and decreases pesticide residues in breast and milk.

TIP: Did you know that tight bras may stop the milk production and cause plugged ducts?

• Cumin helps increase milk production.

• Caraway, aniseed, dill, and fennel promote flow of best milk. It can be taken in form of teas or infusion.

• If you are prone to chills while breast-feeding and have poor quality of milk, use calcarea.

Milk Production Tea.

1 tsp. vitex berries.

1 tsp. blessed thistle leaves.

1/2 tsp. nettle leaves.

1/4 tsp. fenugreek seed.

1/4 tsp. anise seed.

1 quart boiling water.

Mix all ingredients and steep for 20 minutes. Strain and drink 2 cups a day.

Engorgement

Breast engorgement is a very common problem that starts affecting the mother in the first two or three weeks after delivery and is more annoying to women with poor skin elasticity. Engorgement is due to milk excessively filling the breast together with blood and fluid retention in the same area.

Usually the breast feels full, hard, tight, tender, painful, the breast feels hot to the touch and a fever may develop. The baby may also have a hard time to latch on and suck.

We recommend

• Take a handful of Confrey leaves and steam them for a few

minutes wrapped in a gauze. Place on the breast for help in relieving engorgement.

• Take the homeopathic remedy Belladonna 6X.

• Soak a towel in hot water and place it on the breast ten minutes before feeding.

• Poke roots reduce swollen breast and pain. Use under doctor supervision.

• Elder is used to reduce swelling of engorged breast.

• Chamomile helps control inflamed breast.

• Give your baby frequent feeds on both breasts, 10 to 15 minutes each.

• Use a pump to extract milk between feedings to control engorgement.

• Massage the breast while feeding to help milk flow easily.

Mix 2 quarts of boiling water.

2 tsp. of   vitex berries.

2 tsp. of   blessed thistle leaves.

1 tsp. of nettle leaves.

½ tsp. fenugreek seed.

½ tsp. anise seed.

Let it steep for 30 minutes, strain and drink 2 cups a day.

• Bryonia reduces swollen and hard breasts.

• Pulsatilla and calcarea are very helpful reducing the size and hardness of engorged breasts.

• When the production of milk is excessive and produces

engorgement, a cold compress using peppermint oil should be used.

• A compress of marshmallow and slippery elm often reduces engorgement.

Plugged Ducts

This is a problem that occurs when the baby does not empty the breast completely on each feeding. The milk remaining in the duct hardens and blocks the duct eventually plugging it. Tight bras can cause plugged ducts as well. If the breast feels sore, it might be a sign of plugged ducts. A plugged duct should be taken care of as soon as possible, otherwise it can develop into Mastitis.

We recommend

• Castor oil helps with inflammation and pain.

• Elder is used to reduce swelling of plugged breast ducts.

• Queen's Delight clears congestion of lymphatic vessels and, stimulates white blood cells to react to infection.

• Check your nipples every day. If you see dry milk on them or dark dots remove them with a cotton ball and warm water and feed your child as soon as possible from that breast.

• Place the baby in different positions every time. This will ensure that all ducts are being used.

• Place hot towels on the breast or run hot water over them in the shower.

• Massage the breast in the direction of the nipple to try to get the milk to come out.

Mastitis

Mastitis is a condition that results when a plugged duct becomes infected. The breast swells due to some bacteria that enters through tiny cracks on the nipples. The breast infected with mastitis becomes red and painful with pus secretion. Other symptoms are fever, fatigue, vomiting or nausea.

We recommend

• Take poke roots this helps mastitis. Use under doctor supervision.

• Queen's Delight clears congestion of lymphatic vessels, stimulates white blood cells to react to infection.

- Place hot towels on the breast or run hot water over them in the shower.

- Elder is used to reduce swelling of breast infected with mastitis.

- Rest as much as you can.

- Drink lots of water or alfalfa juice.

- Coat your nipples with breast milk after feeding.

- There are antibiotics that are safe for nursing mothers and their babies. See your doctor if your case is very severe. However, we recommend that you try to avoid antibiotics as much as you can.
- Wash your hands before and after feeding to prevent bacterial contamination.

- Dandelion is very helpful and a popular herb to treat mastitis.

- The Chinese use gentian to cure mastitis.

• Madder root is useful in relieving mastitis.

Cracked Nipples

Cracked nipples can develop when the baby is being positioned wrongly or by using damp breast pads. The nipple becomes irritated, red, and painful and in some cases, bleeding may develop.

• Calendula cream will soothe and encourage the healing of cracked nipples and is safe for the baby to swallow.

• The homeopathic remedy called chamomilla helps heal cracked nipples.

• The homeopathic remedy called pulsatilla helps heal cracked nipples.

• Sulfur is also helpful for cracked nipples.

• Apply vitamin E to sore and cracked nipples.

Morning Sickness:

Approximately 50% of all pregnant women experience nausea and vomiting between the sixth and the twelfth week of pregnancy. It's completely normal and can occur at any time of the day although it is called morning sickness. But one in 300 women will have severe abnormal vomiting which is continual nausea and vomiting after the twelfth week. This type of vomiting is called Hiperemesis gravidarum and it can result in dehydration, acidosis, malnutrition and weight loss. This condition can be dangerous to the fetus if it persists. The reason for Hiperemesis gravidarum has not been identified yet but an association between high levels of the hormones estrogen and chronic gonadotropin (HCG) has been found. HCG is a hormone produced by the placenta that increases until the end of the first trimester.

Other possible problems related with abnormal to severe vomiting includes bile duct disease, drug toxicity, pancreatitis, low blood sugar,

71

problems with the thyroid and inflammatory bowel disorders.

In a more natural term, morning sickness is seen as a cleansing of toxins from the system that is preparing for pregnancy.

We recommend :

• Eat frequently during the day (at least six small meals daily) to help you avoid an empty stomach.

• Low blood sugar aggravates the nausea so you should try to keep a good level throughout the day staring from the moment you wake up. You can keep some crackers on your night table and eat them before you get up.

• Instead of eating your foods, try to drink them, it's easier for your body to digest a milk shake or fruit shake instead of having to chew them.

• Avoid foods and odors that make you feel nausea.

• Drink plenty of carbonated beverages without caffeine. Consuming ginger ale for example will promote the elimination of gas. Ginger ale contains ginger, a herb that soothes the digestive tract.

• Also mix single drops of ginger, fennel and peppermint oils, then add them in an ounce of carrier oil. This exquisite oil massaged into the skin will settle the stomach.

• For something more relaxing, put a few drops of lavender oil in the bath tub and enjoy the immersion.

• Taking ½ to 1 tsp of Wild yam root every day will help you deal with your morning sickness.

• A good tea can be made mixing equals parts of two or three of these herbs: Fennel, Cinnamon, Peppermint or Raspberry.

• Another useful tea can be made mixing :

2 tsp Meadowsweet

1 tsp Black Horehound

1 tsp Chamomile

Take a china or glass teapot which has been previously warmed, add one teaspoonful of the dried herb mixture into it for each cup of tea that you intent to brew. After that, pour a cup of boiling water in for each teaspoonful of herb that is already in the pot and then put the lid on. Let it settle for 10 minutes approximately.

• Important•:Infusions may be drunk hot because that is the best way of obtaining results from a medicinal herbal tea. But they can be drunk cold or you can have ice in them if desire. They may be sweetened with honey, brown sugar or Licorice Root.

• During your pregnancy it's important to take the correct vitamins and minerals that will help you and your baby to be healthy. Here are the required during your pregnancy:

Vitamin A: 5,000 IU   Vitamin K: 65 mg

Vitamin B1: 1.5 mg   Folic Acid: 800 mcg

Vitamin B2: 1.6 mg   Calcium: 1,200 mg

Vitamin B3: 17 mg   Magnesium: 500 mg

Vitamin B6: 2.2 mg   Iron: 30 mg

Vitamin B12: 2.2 mcg Phosphorus: 1,200 mg

Vitamin C: 500-1,000 mg   Iodine: 175 mcg

Vitamin D: 400 IU   Selenium: 65 mcg

Vitamin E: 400 IU

In addition take the following vitamins in complement with these:

• Vitamin B6 (25 mg) with Vitamin C (250 mg) and Vitamin K (5 mg) twice daily to prevent morning sickness.

• There is another supplement that you can take to prevent morning sickness which is L-Methionine and the suggested dosage is 1,000 mg daily.

• Next we'll describe some homeopathic remedies:

• If you find yourself vomiting with anxiety and you feel it right into your stomach, or if you can't stand the smell of food because it makes you nausea, you are always very thirsty or in the moment after eating or drinking cold beverages you feel worse, take Arsenicum.

• If right after eating you have sudden spasmodic vomiting and if you see mucous in your vomit, take Antimonium Tartaricum.

• If every time you have nausea or vomits you burp, if you have cravings for sweets and if you feel better outdoors, take Argentrum Nitricum.

• If you don't tolerate the smell or thought of food although you want or feel the necessity of eating them, or you have severe nausea from the sight of food, you feel thirsty and if your condition gets worse every time you move, take Colch.

• If you have the desire to vomit but can't, or your vomit is violent if you are constipated, irritable, or every time you eat your condition gets worse take, Nux Vomica.

• If you vomit but still have good appetite or feel uninterested and fatigued take Sepia.

- If you have nausea, chills and profuse salivation, take Tabacum.

MENOPAUSE

There are also effective natural strategies for preventing or slowing the progression of some of the longer term consequences of estrogen deficiency, such as cardiovascular disease and osteoporosis. Even if you take hormone replacement therapy, dietary modification, nutritional and dietary supplements, herbs, and other naturopathic approaches can be used to great advantage.

NATURAL THERAPIES FOR THE SYMPTOMS OF MENOPAUSE

Many of the discomforts of the menopausal period can be helped with simple, natural treatments that you can use at home, such as increasing your consumption of foods that contain natural plant estrogens, drinking adequate amounts of water, taking selected nutritional supplements, and using specific herbs. Table 6.1 gives an overview of the nutritional and dietary supplements, herbs, and other measures recommended for some of the most common menopausal symptoms.

You can choose to use one, several, or all of the therapies recommended, and you can use these natural treatments either alone or in combination with hormone replacement therapy.

Natural Plant Estrogens

Over 300 different plants contain estrogenic substances. Although these are weak estrogens and are present only in tiny quantities, if foods containing them are consumed regularly, 1 Alfalfa contains a plant estrogen called coumestrol, which can actually cause infertility in animals that graze on large pastures of alfalfa grasses. Of all the plant estrogens, coumestrol is the most potent, although it is still 200 times weaker than human estrogens. The herb red clover also contains coumestrol and can be taken in the form of an herbal tea, or you can make fresh sprouts from red clover seeds. As some varieties of red clover are poisonous, however, it is best to obtain supplies from a reputable herbalist or health food store.

Soybeans, soybean sprouts, and flaxseed meal (crushed flaxseeds) are excellent sources of natural estrogens as well as of protein and essential fatty acids. They are definitely anti-aging foods for menopausal women. For a list of foods and herbs that are good sources of plant estrogens.

Natural plant estrogens provide a useful form of estrogen supplementation for women who are unable to or who choose not to take estrogen replacement therapy. Because these plant estrogens are low in potency, they are safe and will not produce the side effects sometimes seen with HRT. If you want to boost your estrogen level, I suggest you eat approximately two cups daily of foods that we will go into more details later —for example, two cups of mixed sprouts, parsley, soybeans, legumes, and fennel, along with a wide selection of fresh vegetables. Make sure you vary your sources of plant estrogens by using different foods each day to make up your two cups' worth of estrogenic foods.

Plant estrogens are also present in bourbon, whiskey, gin, ouzo, and beer. These estrogens are partly responsible for the breast development seen in alcoholic males, as their damaged livers are unable to break down and inactivate the estrogens found in alcoholic beverages. However, I do not recommend that you try to increase your estrogen level by drinking alcohol.

Table 1 Naturopathic Strategies for Symptoms of Menopause

The following table offers suggestions for herbs, dietary supplements, and other natural strategies that are helpful for common menopausal symptoms. Note that the dosages for some of the items recommended are given in milligrams (mg), some in micrograms (mcg), and some in international units (IU). Both milligrams and micrograms are measures of weight (1 milligram is equal to 1,000 micrograms). International units are measures of the activity of a substance, not its weight; the number of milligrams or micrograms in an international unit therefore varies, depending on the substance being measured. Note also that appropriate doses of herbs may vary depending on the individual; if you have any doubts, consult a qualified herbalist or naturopathic physician for a personalized herbal prescription.

Problem	Strategies
Hot flashes, sweating	Drink (8 glasses) of water daily.
	Take 1,000 mg of evening primrose oil and 100 IU of vitamin E, three times a day.
	Take one or more of the following herbs daily:
	1,000 mg of long quaff
	500-1,000 mg of licorice (or 1-2 cups of licorice tea).
	500-1,000 mg of black cohosh.
	500-1,000 mg of sarsaparilla (or 2-3 cups of sarsaparilla tea).
	300-600 mg of chaste tree (Vitex Agnus-castus).
Dry, Itchy skin	Drink (8 glasses) of water daily.
vaginal dryness	Take 1,000 mg of evening primrose oil.

Note: Licorice can elevate blood pressure. If you have high blood pressure, use it with caution or avoid it entirely.

Problems	Strategies
	Take the following antioxidant supplements (with food):
	5,000 IU of vitamin A or 10 mg of beta-carotene, once daily.
	500 IU of vitamin 8, once daily.
	50 mcg of selenium, once daily.

	1,000-2,000 mg of vitamin C with bioflavonoids, three times daily.
	Use only cold-pressed vegetable oils such as olive, flaxseed, grape seed, canola, and sesame oils in cooking and salad dressings.
Fatigue, poor memory, reduced mental efficiency	Take a balanced high-potency vitamin B complex tablet or capsule daily.
	Take 1,000 mg of evening primrose oil, three times a day.
	Take 1,000 mg of ginkgo biloba, 1,000-4,000 mg of ginseng, and/or 1,000 mg of royal jelly daily.
Anxiety, irritability, mood disorders, insomnia	Take one or more of the following herbs daily (take them at bedtime for insomnia):
	250 mg of passion flower.
	1,000 mg of valerian root (or 2 cups of valerian root tea).
	1-2 cups of lime flower tea.
	1-2 tablespoons of oats.
	500 mg of skullcap.
	Take 4,000 mg of lecithin and 500-1,500 mg of the amino acid L-glutamine daily.
	Take a balanced high-potency vitamin B complex tablet or capsule daily, plus additional amounts of the following:
	500 mg vitamin B5 (pantothenic acid).
	500 mg of choline.
	50 ma of vitamin Bs (pyridoxine).
	Take 500 mg of magnesium (as magnesium cheiate) daily.
Muscle and joint aches and pains, degenerative diseases of the bones, muscles, and joints	Take 1,000 mg of evening primrose oil, three times daily.
	Take 1,000 mg of fish oil daily.
	Take the following antioxidant supplements

	daily:
	10,000 IU of vitamin A or 20 mg of beta-carotene.
	2,000 mg of vitamin C (in mineral ascorbate form with bioflavonoids).
	500 IU of vitamin E.
	Take the following minerals:
	1,000 mg of calcium at bedtime.
	500 mg of magnesium at bedtime.
	1.5-3.0 mg of copper daily.
	20 mg of boron (as sodium borate) daily.
	25 mg of silica daily.
	10 mg of manganese (as manganese chelate) daily
	30 mg of zinc (as zinc chelate) daily.
	400 IU of vitamin Ds (cholecalciferoi) and 100 mcg of vitamin K daily.
Rapid aging of the skin, thinning hair, brittle nails, osteoporosis	Take 1,000 mg of calcium and 500 mg of magnesium at bedtime.
	Take the following vitamins daily:
	5,000 IU of vitamin A or 20 mg of beta-carotene.
	2,000 mg of vitamin C, preferably in mineral ascorbate form with bioflavonoids.
	500 IU of vitamin E.
	400 IU of vitamin D3 (cholecalciferol).
	100 mcg of vitamin K.
	Take the following minerals daily:
	20 mg of boron (as sodium borate).
	5 mg of copper (as copper chelate).
	30 mg of zinc (as zinc chelate).
	25 mg of silica.
	10 mg of manganese (as manganese chelate).

Water and Menopause

Many women find the drinking of pure water a chore and do it grudgingly, much like a penance. It is an acquired habit, but once you start drinking between one and two quarts of pure water daily, your body will soon crave it if you forget. Just think how tired and sad plants look without water. Well, we are just the same!

You may flavor your water with herbal teas or a dash of fresh citrus fruit, but otherwise leave it pure, so that it can act as a cleanser and detoxifier. There is no other cleanser like water. I see many women in their middle years with conditions such as joint pains, bad breath, and osteoarthritis, who did not start drinking adequate amounts of water until it was too late.

Start today. Drink at least one and a half quarts of pure water, gradually, throughout the morning and afternoon. Keep a jug of water on your desk or carry a water bottle with you on your travels. It's well worth the extra trips to the bathroom! By drinking cool water regularly you will reduce hot flashes, headaches, joint pains, fatigue, and dry, itchy skin, and you will rejuvenate your entire cardiovascular system.

Nutritional and Dietary Supplements

There are a number of nutritional and dietary supplements that are especially useful to women who are going through menopause. In addition to supporting overall health, certain nutrients can actually.

Foods Containing Natural Estrogens

A number of different foods and herbs are sources of natural plant estrogens, and can be very helpful during menopause. The following is a list of some of the best food sources of estrogen. These foods not only contain estrogens, but are high in vitamins, minerals, fiber, and essential fatty acids, and they are low in saturated fat. Thus, there are many good reasons to consume them on a regular basis.

Alfalfa

Fennel

Red beans

Anise seed

Flaxseeds Red clover

Apples

Garlic

Rhubarb

Baker's yeast

Green beans

Rice

Barley

Green squash

Rye

Beets

Hops

Sage

Cabbage

Licorice

Sesame seeds

Carrots Oats   Soybean sprouts

Help to relieve unpleasant symptoms. The supplements I recommend include vitamins, minerals, amino acids, and essential fatty acids.

Vitamin A

Vitamin A has many essential roles in the body. It is required for night vision, a healthy immune system, and reproduction. It is also an antioxidant.

Persons lacking in vitamin A may develop skin and mucous membrane disorders in which the tissues become white, hard, and chronically inflamed. This makes them more susceptible to infection.

Vitamin A comes in two forms: preformed vitamin A (retinal or retinyl esters), which is found in cod and halibut liver, cream, butter, eggs, and animal meats and livers; and provitamin A (beta-carotene), which is found in sweet potatoes, papayas, apricots, watermelons, and tomatoes, and in green, yellow, and orange vegetables. The liver converts beta-carotene into vitamin A as the body needs it.

Both vitamin A and beta-carotene strengthen mucous membranes throughout the body. This is helpful for the unpleasant menopausal symptoms of vaginal dryness and fragility. I have found that the combination of vitamin A (or beta-carotene) and evening primrose oil is effective in reducing the itchy, crawling sensation in the skin that often occurs during menopause.

The U.S. recommended daily allowance of vitamin A is 5,000 international units. However, smokers, regular drinkers of alcohol, junk-food consumers, diabetics, and those exposed to excessive pollutants and toxic chemicals often need more. If you have dry and irritated skin and mucous membranes, it is safe to take 10,000 international units of vitamin A or 20,000 to 25,000 international units of beta-carotene daily. Doses above 10,000 international units of vitamin A daily should not be taken without medical supervision, as very high doses (25,000 to

50,000 international units daily) can be toxic. A pregnant woman should never take more than 5,000 international units of vitamin A daily.

Unlike vitamin A, beta-carotene is nontoxic, even in high doses, so there is no need to worry about over dosage. However, no more than 25,000 international units daily is needed to achieve maximal benefits.

The B Vitamins

The B vitamins are a vital group of nutrients that are involved in the functioning of the nervous system and in maintaining healthy skin, eyes, and hair. They also support adrenal gland function and are involved in energy production. The B vitamins should always be taken as a group, in a balanced B complex supplement. If you take any of the B vitamins individually, you should also take a B complex supplement at a different time of day.

Vitamin B5 (pantothenic acid), vitamin B6 (pyridoxine), and choline are three simple and inexpensive nutrients that can neatly provide help for the common menopausal symptoms of anxiety, poor sleep, and loss of libido. Vitamin B6 is required for the conversion of amino acids into neurotransmitters (brain chemicals). In particular, B6 is essential for the conversion of the amino acid tryptophan into the neurotransmitter serotonin. Serotonin exerts an antidepressant effect, and normal amounts are required for a healthy libido. The recommended daily dose of vitamin B6 is 50 to 100 milligrams. Do not take more than this, or transient nerve damage can occur. Good food sources of vitamin B6 are meats, whole grains, and brewer's yeast.

Vitamin B5 and choline are the precursors for the neurotransmitter acetylcholine. Acetylcholine is required for the normal functioning of memory. People who suffer from anxiety often have excessive levels of adrenaline and insufficient amounts of acetylcholine in their bodies.

Acetylcholine is one of the neurotransmitters required for the action of the autonomic nervous system, which is involved in sexual excitement and orgasm. Ensuring adequate levels of acetylcholine helps to maintain sexual responsiveness and enjoyment of lovemaking.

The recommended dose of both vitamin B5 and choline is 500 milligrams daily. Vitamin B5 is present organ meats, eggs, and whole grain cereals. Good food sources of choline include lecithin, eggs, soybeans, cauliflower, cabbage, tofu, and tempeh.

Vitamin C

Vitamin C, or ascorbic acid, is so vital to human health that I have often thought it to be an evolutionary defect that the human body does not manufacture its own supply. Most animals produce their own supplies of vitamin C, which increase when they are under stress.

Vitamin C was made famous by the research of the late Dr. Linus Pauling. Dr. Pauling, twice a Nobel laureate, stated that vitamin C could prevent the common cold and treat cancer. Many doctors believe that vitamin C can reduce the severity of colds and help prevent cancer, although it cannot control established, advanced cancers. Still other doctors do not believe in using nutritional supplements at all—generally because university medical schools are only just starting to include in their curricula any study of nutrition as a therapeutic tool.

Vitamin C is needed for the manufacture of collagen, which acts like a flexible or elastic protein glue in connective tissue and bone. Ensuring plentiful vitamin C helps to maintain healthy collagen, thereby keeping the skin and mucous membranes thicker and stronger and the skeleton more flexible. If your ligaments and bones are more flexible, they are less likely to be torn (sprained) or broken (fractured). Vitamin C is also a powerful antioxidant and free-radical scavenger that helps to reduce degenerative diseases and inflammation, and to slow down the aging process.

Vitamin C is found in high concentrations in the brain and the adrenal glands, and it is required for these organs to function under stress. I always recommend that people who are under mental or physical stress take additional vitamin C, and have found it to have a natural relaxing effect.

The recommended dose of vitamin C is quite a controversial subject among doctors. Although many agree that the U.S. recommended daily allowance of 60 milligrams is inadequate for optimal health, few agree with Dr. Pauling that the daily requirement is between 2,000 and 9,000 milligrams. What is true is that the daily requirement for vitamin C varies greatly among individuals. Factors that increase a person's daily requirement are stress, smoking, infections, surgery, exposure to pollution, and the consumption of alcohol. If you do not eat fresh raw fruits and vegetables every day, you may be deficient in vitamin C, as the body is continually using it up. Vitamin C is destroyed by high temperatures, which is why raw foods are so important.

I believe it is imperative to get at least 1,000 milligrams daily, and if any factors that increase your need, such as those mentioned above, are present, you may require up to 6,000 milligrams daily. It is best to take it in divided doses, with food. However, it is much better to get your vitamin C from natural, fresh raw food sources than to rely on supplements alone. Good food sources of vitamin C include citrus fruits, tomatoes, capsicum, Brussels sprouts, broccoli, berries (blueberries, gooseberries, raspberries, strawberries), bananas, alfalfa, guava, kidney, oysters, potatoes, cantaloupe, sweet potatoes, spinach, watermelon, green leafy vegetables, green and red peppers, sprouted grains, and rose hips.

In most of the high-vitamin-C foods, there are also other nutrients, called bioflavonoids (or, occasionally, vitamin P). There are around 500 different bioflavonoids found in food plants.

Bioflavonoids aid in the absorption and utilization of vitamin C and enhance its antioxidant properties. Some vitamin C supplements contain bioflavonoids as well.

Vitamin D

Vitamin D, or cholecalciferol, functions as both a vitamin and a hormone. Vitamin D is synthesized in the skin when the skin is exposed to the sun's ultraviolet rays. It is required for the absorption and utilization of calcium and helps calcium to be deposited in your bones. Gross deficiencies of vitamin D cause osteomalacia, which is a bone demineralizing disease not unlike osteoporosis.

Osteomalacia is the adult equivalent of childhood rickets. Even marginal or slight deficiencies of vitamin D can increase your risk of osteoporosis and deterioration of the joints. Deficiencies of vitamin D can also contribute to thinning of the hair, brittleness of the nails, and rapid aging of the skin.

Vitamin D is not present in a wide variety of foods, but is confined mainly to fish liver oils, fatty fish, liver, egg yolks, and butter, and, to a lesser degree, cow's milk. It is not unusual for women to be deficient in vitamin D, as many of us now avoid the sun and at the same time, in our constant effort to lose weight, we are reducing the amount of eggs, dairy products, and fatty fish we eat. Those who have difficulty digesting and absorbing fats can easily develop suboptimal levels of vitamin D. Your doctor can test you for vitamin D deficiency with a simple blood test.

The U.S. recommended daily allowance of vitamin D is 400 international units. Supplements of 200 to 400 international units daily are a good idea if you avoid sunlight and fatty foods. Take vitamin D supplements with meals or drink vitamin-D-fortified milk. Do not take excessive doses of vitamin D, however, as this may cause very high blood calcium levels, calcifications in the body's soft tissues and organs, and kidney stones. Doses less than 1,000 international units daily are considered most unlikely to exert any dangerous effects. Even so, if you have a tendency to develop kidney stones, you should take vitamin D or calcium supplements only under medical supervision.

Vitamin E

Vitamin E is essential for the existence of all oxygen-breathing creatures. It has a protective, or sparing, effect on estrogen, so that your estrogen (whether your own or from hormone replacement therapy) lasts longer. As a result, vitamin E helps to reduce hot flashes. Some women have told me that vitamin E supplements delayed menopause and the state of estrogen deficiency. Perhaps the ancient Greeks knew of the hormonal benefits of eating foods high in vitamin E; the chemical name for vitamin E is tocopherol, which in Greek means "to carry and bear babies."

Together with vitamin A, vitamin E strengthens the skin and mucous membranes. Many women find that these vitamins reduce vaginal dryness and shrinkage. Vitamin E also reduces free radical damage to your cells' membranes and is a poweful anti-aging nutrient.

The recommended daily dose of vitamin E is from 100 to 500 international units daily. Start slowly, gradually building up the dosage, to avoid a sudden boost to your cardiovascular system. Over the long term, daily doses of 100 international units are generally sufficient. If you find brown age spots appearing on your skin, taking additional vitamin E can reverse this degenerative process. Take 500 international units daily until the spots fade, and apply a combination of vitamin E cream and aloe vera gel to the affected areas twice daily.

Vitamin K

Vitamin K is a fat-soluble vitamin that is needed for the synthesis of several blood-clotting factors, and for this reason it can reduce the heavy menstrual bleeding that is common in the perimenopausal years. Vitamin K is also needed for the mineralization of bone and helps to keep your bones stronger and more resilient to breakage. Some preliminary studies suggest

that vitamin K can be significant in the prevention of osteoporosis.

Vitamin K deficiency is not common, as this nutrient is present in many different types of foods, and bacteria in the intestines synthesize a large proportion of daily vitamin K requirements. If you take antibiotics frequently, however, you can greatly reduce your production of vitamin K. A tendency to bruise easily can be a sign of vitamin K deficiency.

The recommended daily allowance for vitamin K is 65 micrograms, an amount that normally is easily obtained in the diet. Good food sources include green leafy vegetables, egg yolks, blackstrap molasses, alfalfa, kelp, nettles, dairy products, wheat bran, wheat germ, soybean oil, and cod liver oil. Foods containing lactobacillus bacteria (such as kefir, whey, and yogurt) add friendly bacteria that produce vitamin K to the intestines. If you have malabsorption or digestive problems, or take antibiotics frequently, a supplement of 50 to 100 micrograms daily is desirable.

Boron

Boron is a trace mineral found in plant foods, and its health benefits are becoming increasingly evident. A study done in 1987 found that boron may be helpful in preventing osteoporosis?

Twelve postmenopausal women between the ages of forty-eight and eighty-two were studied for twenty-four weeks. During the first seventeen weeks, they were given a diet low in boron (which is what many women normally consume), and during the subsequent seven weeks they received 3 milligrams of boron daily.

Eight days after they began taking boron, the wornen's urinary losses of calcium and magnesium were greatly reduced, and they had significant increases (approximately twofold) in their production of estrogen and testosterone. Reducing the loss of magnesium from the body is very desirable, as magnesium is essential for a healthy cardiovascular system and skeleton. This research suggests that taking boron supplements, especially if your dietary intake of boron is low, can cause favorable changes in mineral metabolism that can reduce, and may even prevent, the loss of mineral from the bones (osteoporosis). Boron is also necessary for healthy hair, skin, and nails, and an adequate intake of boron may help prevent muscle and joint aches and pains.

Foods high in boron include fruits, vegetables, and sesame seeds. Meats and poultry, on the other hand, are low in boron. Boron is available in supplement form, most commonly as sodium borate. An appropriate dosage would be 5 to 20 milligrams daily.

Calcium

As discussed in Chapter 2, many perimenopausal women do not consume the recommended daily allowance of 1,000 milligrams of calcium. This can increase their risk of developing osteoporosis, cardiovascular disease, arthritis, cramps, and fragile skin. Calcium and magnesium work together to form bone substance and to regulate muscular tone, and they are required in a ratio of 2 to i (that is, 200 milligrams of calcium per 100 milligrams of magnesium). Every woman should consume at least 1,000 milligrams of calcium per day, either from food sources or in supplement form.

Copper

Copper is an essential trace mineral. Together with iron, copper enables the blood protein hemoglobin to carry precious oxygen to your cells.

Copper is a component in superoxide dismutase, an antioxidant enzyme produced by the body that protects against damage from free radicals. Copper is bound to the protein ceruloplasmin, which is a very important antioxidant in the blood. Ceruloplasmin prevents peroxidation (rancidity) of the polyunsaturated fats in cell membranes. An adequate intake of copper is also needed for healthy skin, hair, nails, and bones. It is involved in the production of collagen, a tough, fibrous, yet elastic, tissue found in bone, tendons, skin, and cartilage. Indeed, copper is a known folk remedy for arthritis; some people swear by their copper bracelets.

Symptoms of copper deficiency include anemia, osteoporosis, and brittle, inflexible bones.

There is a wide variation in dietary copper intake, and many women may be getting sub-optimal amounts. This may not cause obvious symptoms, but it is a concern, given copper's vital role in maintaining bone and ligament integrity and in forming antioxidant reserves.

Good food sources of copper are animal liver, crustaceans, nuts, oysters, legumes, kidneys, fruits, and shellfish. You can also take copper in supplement form, as copper gluconate, copper sulfate, or copper amino acid chelate. The recommended dose is 1.5 to 3 milligrams daily. The ratio of copper to zinc taken in supplement form should be 1 to 10; that is, if you take 30 milligrams of zinc, then the required dose of copper is 3 milligrams. However, if you have Wilson's disease—a rare hereditary syndrome characterized by an inability to metabolize copper properly—you should not take any copper supplements.

Magnesium

Magnesium is a mineral that has many important functions in the body. Among other things, it is involved in the production of enzymes and in the process by which cellular energy is released. Because it plays an important role in regulating muscular tone, it can serve as a natural muscle relaxant, making it useful for relieving such symptoms as muscle cramping and anxiety. Many menopausal women suffer from heart palpitations (an irregular or racing heartbeat) associated with hot flashes. This can be helped by increasing your intake of magnesium. Magnesium and calcium supplementation, in a ratio of 2 milligrams of calcium for each milligram of magnesium, can reduce bone loss after menopause. Magnesium is also essential for the health of the heart and the circulatory system. An appropriate supplemental dose of magnesium is around 500 milligrams daily.

Manganese

Manganese is a vital mineral for health and is required for the metabolism of food and the production of sex hormones. Like copper, it is an antioxidant and is an element in superoxide dismutase, a potent antioxidant enzyme, and thus helps to reduce degenerative diseases associated with aging. Manganese is also part of normal bone and cartilage structure, and can be helpful for sufferers of osteoarthritis. Some studies have found that women with osteoporosis have low levels of manganese compared with women whose bones are normal.

The National Research Council of America states that an adequate daily intake of manganese is 2 to 5 milligrams, and that up to 10 milligrams daily is safe. Good food sources of manganese are whole grains and nuts, wheat bran, organ meats, shellfish and milk. Many fruits and vegetables contain moderate amounts, but this varies depending on the manganese content of the soil where they were grown. Manganese can be taken in supplement form as manganese gluconate or manganese amino acid chelate.

Selenium

Selenium is a trace mineral that is vital for good health. It is important in maintaining healthy immune function and tissue elasticity, including that of the skin and mucous membranes. It is also an important antioxidant that works synergistically with vitamin E to prevent free radical damage and support the health of the heart and circulatory system.

Silica

Silica is a form of the mineral silicon, -which is the second most abundant element in the earth's outer layer. Silicon is used to make glass and computer chips, among other things, and in the last decade has been found to be an essential trace mineral for animals and for humans.

Silicon is found in human bone, fingernails, skin, and connective tissue, and adds mechanical integrity and hardness to their architectural matrix. Some researchers believe that silicon may offer some protection against atherosclerosis by strengthening connective tissue in the blood vessel walls.

The best food sources of silicon and silica are seafoods, whole grains, and vegetables. If you consume a balanced diet, you probably get about 200 milligrams of silica daily. The herb horsetail is high in silica, and can be taken as a tea or in the form of an extract called vegetal silica. Silica can also be taken as part of a multimineral formula. Taking moderate amounts of supplemental silica has no known side effects. The recommended dosage is 25 to 100 milligrams daily.

Zinc

Zinc is an essential mineral for the body, as more than 200 enzymes require zinc for their activity. It is also important for the proper functioning of cell membranes. Zinc is vital for a healthy immune system and helps to keep hair, nails, and bones strong.

Good food sources of zinc include brewer's yeast, seafoods, whole grain products, wheat bran, lean meats, blackstrap molasses, liver, sesame and sunflower seeds, and oatmeal. Zinc can also be taken in supplement form as zinc amino acid chelate. Recommended supplemental doses for women are 15 to 30 milligrams daily. To avoid possible stomach upset, take zinc supplements with food, and do not exceed the recommended dosage, as the consumption of too much zinc may upset the balance of other necessary minerals in the body. It is best to take zinc on an intermittent basis, for example, three months on, three months off.

L-Glutamine

L-glutamine is an amino acid that crosses the blood-brain barrier and passes into the brain tissue, where it is converted into glutamic acid. The brain then converts glutamic acid into the neurotransmitter gamma-amino-butyric-acid (GABA). GABA is a neuroinhibitory transmitter that regulates many aspects of brain function. Around one third of all the nerve cells in the brain send inhibitory, rather than accelerating, signals, and this is done via GABA.

Taking L-glutamine increases the production of GABA. This process can also be aided synergistically by taking 50 milligrams of vitamin B6daily. Increased levels of GABA in the brain serve as a natural calming and memory-enhancing agent, and generally help one to think more dearly. L-glutamine is also useful for people who tend to use alcohol to help them cope with stress, as it reduces the craving for alcohol.

The recommended dosage of L-glutamine is 500 milligrams, twice daily. L-glutamine should be taken on an empty stomach, preferably with fruit juice.

Royal Jelly

Royal jelly is a natural food supplement that is rich in many essential vitamins, minerals, enzymes, hormones, and amino acids. It also contains antibiotic components. Royal jelly has energy-boosting properties, making it useful for symptoms of fatigue as well as for improving memory and overall mental and physical functioning.

Essential Fatty Acids

The health benefits of essential fatty acids are huge and diverse, and could be the subject of an entire book. Essential fatty acids (EFAs) are vital for the production and release of many hormones, including sex hormones and adrenal hormones. They are also an integral part of cell membranes, and they give these membranes the proper flexibility and suppleness: They stop your cells from drying out and give them normal cohesiveness.

There are two basic types of EFAs, known as omega-3 and omega-6. These nutrients can help overcome dry and/or itchy skin, dry hair, hair loss, dry eyes, and dry mouth, and can reduce vaginal dryness. They also help to reduce infections of the skin and mucous membranes such as cystitis, vaginitis, and mouth ulcers.

Many women use expensive creams and shampoos; to no avail; their skin and hair remain unhealthy. This is because they are lacking in EFAs. If you feed your skin and hair from within by using EFAs, you will be delighted with the difference—but give it time. It usually takes three to four months to see results.

Other benefits of EFAs include an improvement in the functioning of the nervous system, so I recommend them for women with a poor memory, insomnia, or mood disorders. Many women find that EFAs have the added benefit of reducing hot flashes, presumably because EFAs enhance and balance the production of sex hormones and prostaglandins. EFAs exert an anti-inflammatory effect and can reduce the pain of arthritis and general muscular aches and pains.

Essential fatty acids must be obtained from foods like fish, fish oils, and unprocessed fresh vegetables, seeds, nuts, and botanical oils. To boost your intake of omega-6 EFAs, take 2,000 to 3,000 milligrams of evening primrose oil, 1,000 milligrams of lecithin, and 1,000 milligrams of spirulina daily. To increase your level of omega-3 EFAs, take 1,000 to 2,000 milligrams of fish oil capsules daily or increase your consumption of fish to four servings weekly. In addition, use one tablespoon of cold-pressed canola, olive, or sunflower oil in your salad daily. Another tasty way to boost your levels of EFAs at breakfast time is to grind a mixture of flaxseeds, almonds, and sunflower seeds and sprinkle it on your cereal or rice.

Herbs

There are many herbs that contain plant estrogens or that act to stimulate the production of your natural hormones. These herbs can "bridge the gap" between the time when your ovaries cease their estrogen-producing function and when your adrenal glands start producing a different form of estrogen, called estrone. Estrone is not as powerful as the estrogen produced by the ovaries, which is called estradiol; however, it is often enough to reduce unpleasant symptoms during this transition period.

Table 2 lists herbs that are suitable for use in menopause, with a brief overview of their actions, as well as information on how to use them. Herbs can be purchased from health food outlets or from a qualified herbalist.

The appropriate method of preparing an herbal remedy from fresh herbs depends on which part of the plant is used. The flowers and leaves of herbs may be prepared by making a tea.

Bring water to a boil on top of the stove. While the water is boiling, place the herbs in a glass or ceramic (not metal) teapot that has a tight-fitting lid. Use one-half ounce (approximately one tablespoon) of the dried herb to one cup of water. When the water boils, pour it over the herbs, cover, and let the tea steep for ten to fifteen minutes. Then strain it and drink. You can sweeten the tea with a teaspoon of honey if needed.

If you are using the dried root, seeds, or woody parts of a plant, you will need to make what is called a decoction. Place one-half ounce (about one tablespoon) of the dried herb in a glass or enamel (not metal) saucepan and add one cup of cold water. Let the herbs soak in the water for ten minutes, then cover the pot and bring it to a boil over high heat. Reduce the heat and let the mixture simmer for fifteen minutes. Then remove the pot from the heat and let the mixture steep for another ten minutes. Strain it and drink it warm.

Whether you are using a tea or a decoction, I recommend that a cupful be taken warm, not hot, three times a day.

If you do not have the time or inclination to prepare your own herbal teas, you may take herbs in dried form as tablets or capsules. Herbs are also available in the form of tinctures, which are liquid extracts, and as dried extracts, which can be turned into tablets and capsules. Both tinctures and dried extracts are concentrated sources of herbs, so smaller amounts are required to achieve the same effect. In general, I recommend that herbs be taken in tea, tablet, or capsule form, rather than as tinctures, because tinctures contain varying concentrations of the active ingredient, they tend to be very strong- tasting, and they contain alcohol. Consult a qualified herbalist, an herb shop, or your local health food store for availability and for good,

Herbs for Menopause

There are many medicinal herbs that can be helpful for the menopausal woman. This table lists those herbs that I have found to be most valuable, together with their actions and uses. These herbs should be available through an herbalist or at better health food stores.

Herb	Part Used	Actions and Uses
Black cohosh	Dried roots	This is a good estrogenic herb that acts(Chnicifuga racemosa) and rhizomes specifically on the uterus to reduce cramps and congestion. It is also good for relievinghot flashes. Bieck cohosh contains two antirheumatic agents and it is an excellent herb for relieving muscular pain and cramping. It may also help to reduce cholesterol levels and blood pressure. Take

		250 mg in tablet or capsule form, two to four times daily. Or take 1/2 teaspoon of tincture, twice daily.
Chaste tree Vitex agnuscastus)	Dried fruit	This herb is a hormone balancer that is used to alleviate depression at menopause. Take 300-600 mg in tablet or capsule form daily. Or take 1/2 teaspoon of tincture, twice daily. Darniana (Turners offlosa)Dried leaves Damiana Is a great herb for menopause because it is a pituitary regulator and antidepressant. It is also an aphrodisiac and is of benefit for sexual difficulties. It should not be taken too frequently, however, or it may irritate the lining of the urinary tract; I recommend taking 100-150 mg in tablet or capsule form; for two or three days out of the week. Or take 1/2 teaspoon of tincture, twice daily, for two or three days out of the week.
Dandelion	Leaves , roots	Dandelion is a wonderful herb for the liver. If your hormones are out of balance, then your liver is under extra stress, and dande-lion root will be beneficial for this. Take 1,000-3,000 mg in tablet or capsule form, or 2-3 cups of tea, daily. Or take 1-2 teaspoons of dandelion tincture. Three times daily.
Dong quai (Angelica sinensis)	Roots	This herb is high in natural plant estrogens called phytosterols and helps to reduce the symptoms of estrogen deficiency. Take 500 mg in tablet or capsule form, twice daily. Or take 1/2 teaspoon of tincture, twice daily.
False unicorn root	Dried roots	This plant is an estrogen regulator. It has a direct action on the uterus and ovaries and is considered to be a corrective herb for women. It is a specific for the herbal

		treatment of ovarian cysts. Take 500 mg in tablet or capsule form, or 1 teaspoon of tincture, daily.
Ginkgo Biloba	Leaves	This herb improves brain function, circulation, oxygenation of all body cells. it is helpful for symptoms of fatigue, memory problems, and depression. Take 1,000 mg in tablet or capsule form daily. Or take 1 teaspoon of tincture, twice daily.
Ginseng	Roots	Ginseng strengthens the adrenal glands, enhances immune function, increases energy,and normalizes blood pressure. It is useful for senticosus, symptoms of both mental and physical fatigue.
Panax quinque	folios	Take 1,000-4,000 mg in tablet or capsule form daily. Ginseng is a safe energy-booster for most people. However, if you have very high blood pressure (over 180/100), you should avoid it. Siberian ginseng appears to be more effective than the American variety.
Licorice	Dried roots rhizomes	Licorice is a powerful adrenal stimulant and is a wonderful estrogenic herb. For this reason, it is a very useful herb during menopause. Care must be taken, however, not to take licorice too often, or it can deplete potassium and elevate blood pressure. If you have high blood pressure, use it with caution or avoid it entirely. On the other hand, if you suffer from low blood pressure, this herb will be useful in correcting the problem. Licorice makes a pleasant-tasting tea. It can also be added in small amounts to other herbal teas to improve their flavor. For hot flashes, I recommend drinking 1-2

		cups of licorice tea or taking 500-1,000 mg in tablet or capsule form daily. Or take 1/2-1 teaspoon of tincture, twice daily.
Raspberry (Hubusictaeus)	Fresh or dried leaves	Raspberry Is an astringent and nutritive estro genic herb. It has a direct action on the muscles and fruit of the uterus, helps to tone weakened uterine muscles, and relaxes uterine and intestinal spasms. It also assists In correcting prolapse of the uterus and/or vagina. Take 2,000 mg in tablet or capsule form, or drink 2-3 glasses of raspberry tea daily. Or take 1/2-1 teaspoon of raspberry tincture, up to three times daily.
Red clover	Dried flower	Red clover contains a plant estrogen called coumestrol and one of its medicinal actions is to stimulate the ovaries. It is a good "alkalinizing" herb that is described in herbals as an alternative, which means that it restores healthy body functions. Red clover is a specific for the herbal treatment of ovarian cysts. To relieve hot flashes, take 1,000-2,000 mg of red clover in tablet or capsule form or drink 3-4 cups of red clover tea daily. Or take 1/2- 11/2 teaspoons of red clover tincture, up to three times daily.
Sage or Salvia	Fresh, dried leaves	This herb has many medicinal properties and is very useful during menopause for the Treatment of hot flashes. Sage reduces excessive sweating and it contains plant estrogens. You will find sage particularly helpful in eliminating night sweats. Drink 3-4 cups of sage tea daily to relieve hot flashes, or take 1/2-1 teaspoon of tincture, three times a day. Sprinkle finely

		chopped fresh sage In soups and on salads and vegetables.
St. Johnswort	Fresh or dried flower	This herb is a mild sedative that is specific for anxiety states. It may also be useful for combating in depression. Take 500 mg in tablet or capsule form, or 14-1 teaspoon of tincture, two or three
Sarsaparilla	Dried roots	Sarsaparilla is another alterative herb that stimulates the production of testosterone and therefore improves a flagging libido. It also helps to increase energy. Take 1,000-2,000 mg in tablet or capsule form or drink 2-3 glasses of sarsaparilla tea daily. Or take 1/4-1/2 teaspoon of tincture, up to three times daily.
Saw palmetto	Dried fruit	This herb is an astringent diuretic that is beneficial for the treatment of urinary incontinence, fluid retention, and prolapse of the pelvic organs. Dryness and lack of tone in the tissues of the bladder often lead to irritation and weakness. This is reduced by saw palmetto. This herb can also be useful for combatting chronic urinary tract infection. Take 1,000-2,000 mg in tablet or capsule form daily. Or take 1/2 teaspoon of tincture, twicedaily.

STRATEGIES FOR HEALTHY BLOOD VESSELS

Naturopathic medicine is useful not only for treating the acute discomforts of the perimenopausal period, but also has a role to play in preventing or reducing some of the health problems that result from the lack of estrogen over the long term, after menopause, women are at significant risk of heart and blood vessel disease. Indeed, cardiovascular disease is the number-one killer of women in Western societies, claiming twice as many lives every year as cancer. Although these diseases tend to attack women later than men, this should not stop women from looking for ways to decrease their risk. Furthermore, the survival rate for women who suffer heart attacks is lower than that for men, regardless of age.

Let us take a look at some of the nutritional strategies you can use to decrease your risk of cardiovascular disease. These good nutritional habits will also reduce your risk of cancer and obesity.

Minimize Fats

Reducing the amount of fat in your diet will lower your risk of heart disease and cancer.

Fats and oils are extremely high in calories, and if you eat excessive amounts of them, they slow down your metabolic rate, keeping you from losing weight and contributing to obesity.

One basic principle that will help to cut the amount of fat in your diet is to cut down on meat and dairy products and to increase the proportion of your diet that consists of grains, legumes, fruits, and vegetables. This will also take a load off your kidneys and help you retain calcium. Another way to lessen the amount of fat in your diet is to stop buying processed foods such as packaged cookies, cakes, pastries, and fried foods, which are high in fat.

Avoid frying your foods (especially deep-frying!) and roasting or baking meats in their own fat. Broiling, boiling, steaming, and dry- baking are better. The one exception to this rule is stir-frying, which can be done with a minimum of added oil in a non-stick, non-aluminum pan. When you must use oil, use small amounts of cold-pressed vegetable oils such as canola, olive, sunflower, or grapeseed, and cook your food slowly, at lower temperatures, to avoid having the oil become oxidized. Resist the temptation to add salt or use prepackaged sauces; instead, flavor your foods with vegetable extracts, tomato purée, herbs, and spices.

When you select a prepared food product such as breakfast cereal, take the time to read the product information on the packaging. You may be surprised to find that some popular brands have very high levels of fat, salt, and sugar. Good low-fat alternatives to processed breakfast cereals are oatmeal and natural, unsweetened muesli, as well as barley and brown rice, which can be boiled and eaten as a hot cereal with the addition of a little low-fat milk.

You can also make an excellent mixture called LSA (for linseeds-sunflower seeds-almonds) that can be added to your breakfast cereal. Mix 11/2 cups of linseeds (flaxseeds), 1 cup of sunflower seeds, and 1/2 cup of almonds together and grind them into a fine meal in a food processor or grinder. LSA is an excellent concentrated source of omega-6 essential fatty acids, fiber, natural plant estrogens, protein, calcium, selenium, vitamin E, vitamin A, and the B vitamins. It must be kept fresh; store it in the refrigerator. Start making healthy choices and feel the benefits.

Saturated Fats

When reducing the amount of fat in your diet, it is important to know that all fat is not created equal. In particular, saturated fats are the most important ones to eliminate, as consuming excessive amounts of them can lead to obesity, clogged arteries, and an increased risk of cancer of the breast, ovaries, uterus, and bowel. The most identifiable feature of saturated fats is that they are solid at room temperature.

Examples of saturated fats are the fats found in beef, pork, lamb, poultry, cheese, chocolate, butter, copha, suet, and lard. Meat drippings, whole milk, cream, ice cream, and coconut and palm oils also contain saturated fats. I am not saying that you must avoid these foods completely, but you should keep your consumption of them to as low a level as possible. Make sure that you remove all the fat from meat and the skin from chicken, and use low-fat dairy products. You may eat as much as two to three servings of red meat per week, provided you remove all the fat. Never fry red meat or chicken; bake or broil these meats or use them in casseroles and stews.

Eggs may be eaten in moderation, up to four per week. Eggs contain cholesterol, but they also are an excellent source of the sulfur-containing amino acids L-cysteine and L- methionine. L-cysteine contains a form of sulfur that inactivates free radicals and thus protects and preserves cells It is also a precursor of glutathione, which is a major antioxidant in the body. L-methionine helps to eliminate fatty substances that can otherwise clog the blood vessels, and it is vital for efficient liver function, which helps to rid the body of toxins. The sulfur-containing amino acids found in eggs can thus be considered anti-aging foods. Always boil or poach your eggs, rather than frying them; when fried, eggs produce oxycholesterol, or oxidized cholesterol, a dangerous fat that generates free radical production in the body.

Processed or delicatessen meats, such as processed luncheon meats, smoked or pressed ham, salami, and pepperoni, are not healthy to eat, as they are loaded with saturated fats.

Moreover, because they are not fresh, their fats may become rancid. Rancid fats are highly oxidized and generate free radicals in the body that attack blood vessels and body cells. Also, these meat products contain nitrites, which have been linked to the development of cancer.

Cholesterol

Cholesterol is a pearly fatlike substance that is produced in your liver. It cannot dissolve in water or blood, so it is transported in the bloodstream by specialized molecules called lipoproteins. Lipoproteins are not found in foods, but are manufactured by the liver, and they come in two basic types: high-density lipoproteins (HDL) and low-density lipoproteins (LDL), HDLs are scavengers that pick up free cholesterol in the blood and carry it back to the liver to be reused or broken down. LDLs are larger than HDLs and are heavily laden with cholesterol, which they transport to the body's cells, as needed.

Cholesterol is actually a necessary substance, and if you do not eat any foods that contain it, your body will make it. It becomes a problem, however, when there is more of it present than your body can cope with. Thus, if your diet contains a lot of cholesterol, it may end up being deposited on the walls of your arteries, leading to hardening and blockage of the arteries. To prevent this, it is necessary to have enough HDL circulating in your bloodstream to scavenge excess cholesterol and prevent it from causing harm. You can increase your levels of beneficial high-density lipoproteins by exercising regularly, reducing the amount of saturated fats in your diet, maintaining a healthy weight, and not smoking.

Your body can produce all the cholesterol you need without the need for added dietary cholesterol. If you consume very little dietary cholesterol, your need for high-density lipoproteins will also be low. Generally, it is ideal to have a cholesterol level of less than 200 milligrams per deciliter of blood (200 mg/dL). In some people, elevated blood cholesterol may increase the risk of heart disease. Cholesterol is found mostly in foods of animal origin, such as meat, poultry, seafood, eggs, and dairy products. However, it is not only the amount of cholesterol but also the amount of saturated fats in the diet that affects a person's blood cholesterol level. This is because, when excessive amounts of saturated fats are eaten, the body responds by converting the fat into cholesterol. Foods high in saturated fats include all land animal products such as fatty meats, preserved meats, and whole-milk dairy foods; other sources are shellfish and coconut and palm oils.

Reducing dietary saturated fat is very important, but it is only one of the methods of reducing cholesterol levels. You must also increase your consumption of foods that help to lower cholesterol. These include oily fish (such as salmon, sardines, and tuna), vitamin-C-rich foods (citrus fruits, melons, cabbage, fresh green leafy vegetables, kiwi fruit, sweet and chili peppers, and strawberries), garlic, onions, and foods containing soluble fiber. Soluble fiber is fiber that dissolves easily in water and is found in the gums, pectin, and mucilages of plant fiber. Good sources of soluble fiber are legumes, cereals, whole grains, oat bran, fruits, and vegetables. Soluble fiber protects against gallstones, ulcerative colitis, high blood pressure, high blood cholesterol, and diabetes.

Unsaturated Fats

Unsaturated fats are fats that are liquid at room temperature. Examples are fish oils and olive, flaxseed, canola, grape seed, peanut, corn, safflower, sesame, soybean, and sunflower oils.

These oils are combinations of monounsaturated and polyunsaturated oils. The best choices among these oils are olive, canola, and flaxseed. This is because these oils contain large amounts of monounsaturated oils. Research has shown that these oils can be beneficial to the health of our arteries.3 Mediterranean peoples have consumed these oils regularly for centuries, and have very low rates of heart disease.

Try to obtain cold-pressed vegetable and seed oils, as no fat or oil is healthy if it is subjected to heat processing or if food is fried in it. Both animal fats and vegetable oils, when they are heated to high temperatures, form chemicals that attack and destroy blood vessel walls.

If you use butter or margarine, do so only in moderation (if you are trying to lose weight, it is best to avoid these products altogether). Butter is a natural product, but it is high in cholesterol, saturated fat, and calories. Margarine is a synthetic product that is made by subjecting vegetable oils to a process called hydrogenation. This is what makes margarines solid or semisolid at room temperature. However, hydrogenation also results in the creation of substances called cis- and trans-fatty acids. Cis- and trans-fatty acids are not useful utritional substances and, if consumed regularly in large amounts, can have negative effects on your cardiovascular system. In addition, many brands of margarine contain other added chemicals to make them look and taste more like butter. Thus, while some people once thought that margarine was a healthy alternative to butter, it is now known that a small amount of butter is probably better for you than any amount of margarine. I recommend that you use a spread like tahini, avocado, or hummus instead of either margarine or butter.

Cut Down on Salt

Salt is a compound of two elements, sodium and chloride. Standard table salt consists of 40 percent sodium and 60 percent chloride. Our nutritional requirement for sodium is only 250 to 350 milligrams each day. One level teaspoon of salt contains 2,000 milligrams of sodium, so it is easy to see that many of us eat too much salt. Excess salt in the diet increases your risk of developing high blood pressure, cardiovascular disease, fluid retention, and osteoporosis.

Many menopausal women consume too much sodium. This is not surprising when you consider how much salt is added to processed and convenience foods, and that the salt and pepper shakers are standard additions to the dinner table.

Percentages of Fatty-Acids in Different Oils

Oils from vegetables, seeds, and nuts contain different mixtures of saturated, monounsaturated, and polyunsaturated fats. It is the chemical structure of a fatty acid that determines which class it belongs to. The consumption of saturated fats tends to raise cholesterol levels and has been linked to obesity, heart disease, and a number of different types of cancer. On the other hand, oils high in monounsaturated fatty acids, such as olive, canola, and avocado oil, are beneficial in that they can lower total cholesterol levels. Polyunsaturated fats are sources of essential fatty acids.

There are several things you should do to reduce your sodium intake. Read labels on processed foods and avoid products that contain salt or sodium in any form. Watch for "hidden" sodium, in the form of flavor enhancers and preservatives, such as monosodium glutamate (MSG), hydrolyzed proteins, autolyzed yeast, sodium caseinate, and calcium caseinate. Occasionally, MSG is included in salt shakers at fast food outlets or used to add a different flavor to French fries or chicken; it is a well-known addition to Chinese food. Other label terms that may indicate the presence of sodium in processed foods include malt flavoring, high-flavored yeast, yeast extract, soybean extract, textured soy protein, and even such harmless-sounding terms as "spices" or "seasonings." Artificial sweeteners can also contain high levels of sodium. Reducing your intake of processed and fast foods usually leads to a large reduction of dietary sodium levels.

Finally, stop adding salt to your cooking and put away the salt shaker! At first you will miss the salty taste. You may have strong cravings for salt for even the first few months, but they will pass.

Eventually, your taste buds will readjust and you will be able to taste the more subtle natural flavors of foods again.

Nutritional Supplements for a Healthy Heart

Vitamin A, vitamin C, vitamin E, beta-carotene, and choline, and the minerals zinc and selenium, are known as the antioxidant nutrients. They help to reduce damage to the blood vessels caused by free radicals. (For information about free radicals and antioxidants, see Chapter 7). If possible, find a good-quality antioxidant tablet containing all of these nutrients. If not, you can take each

component separately. I recommend that you take the following daily:

- 10,000 international units of vitamin A or 20 milligrams of beta-carotene.

- 4,000 milligrams of vitamin C with bioflavonoids.

- 100 to 500 international units of vitamin E.

- 30 milligrams of zinc chelate.

- 500 milligrams of choline.

- 50 micrograms of selenium.

Vitamin E is required for energy production and enables muscle cells to use oxygen (the fuel for energy) more efficiently. It is thus beneficial for athletic people and for those wanting to reduce symptoms of heart disease, such as angina and palpitations. Vitamin E reduces oxidant damage to LDL cholesterol and the blood vessel walls, thereby helping to keep your arteries unclogged and your blood flowing freely.

A study conducted at Boston's Brigham and Women's Hospital and the Harvard School of Public Health showed that daily supplementation with vitamin E in doses of 100 to 400 international units reduced the risk of heart attack by 25 to 50 percent in both men and women.

Garlic is the most popular food herb in the world today. It contains selenium, and allicin, which exert beneficial effects on the blood vessels and the immune system. It acts as a natural body cleanser and antibiotic. Best of all, it reduces levels of I.DL (the so-called "bad cholesterol") and reduces the tendency to form blood clots. You may eat garlic fresh or cooked in food, or take odorless garlic capsules; 1,000 to 2,000 milligrams (one to two grams) daily is a suitable dose.

Magnesium is a mineral that is vital for heart muscle relaxation and that improves metabolic 4 sources of magnesium are wheat germ, nuts, soybeans, legumes, whole grains, all dark-green vegetables, and milk. You can also take magnesium tablets. Recommended doses are 400 to 800 milligrams daily.

The herbs ginkgo biloba and bilberry contain bioflavonoids that have a vitamin-C-like action and strengthen the capillaries (tiny blood vessels) in your cardiovascular system.

They are available in tablet or capsule form at pharmacies and health food stores. You can take from 1,000 to 2,000 milligrams of ginkgo biloba and up to 1,000 milligrams of bilberry daily. The supplement coenzyme Qio also plays an important role in energy production in the heart, brain, and body muscles. I recommend a daily dose of 100 to 200 milligrams.

FOODS FOR HEALTHY BONES

Osteoporosis, one of the most serious long-term consequences of estrogen deficiency, is common among postmenopausal women, but it is not inevitable. Good nutrition, especially the consumption of adequate amounts of calcium and other minerals, has an important part to play in both preventing and in slowing the progression of this disease.

Generally speaking, for healthy bones, women require 800 to 1,000 milligrams of calcium daily.

During pregnancy, lactation, and menopause, calcium needs increase to 1,000 to 1,500 milligrams daily.

Good food sources of calcium include dairy products, salmon, tuna, sardines (with the bones), green leafy vegetables, and tofu. Table 6.4 lists foods that are good sources of calcium. Use it to see if your daily diet provides you with an adequate amount of calcium. If your diet falls short of this, or if you are not sure, take a good-quality calcium tablet to give you 1,000 milligrams of calcium daily.

One of the best food sources of calcium is milk, A cup of milk daily will give you a good start to meeting your calcium requirements. When it comes to cow's milk, I recommend calcium-enriched milk, such as Borden's Hi-Calcium or Viva with extra calcium, which is low in fat and much higher in calcium than skim milk. If you are on a dairy-free diet, you may choose calcium-enriched soy milk instead. Some soy milks are calcium enriched; while others are low in calcium, so read labels to be sure the product you choose is a good source of calcium.

There are a number of different supplemental sources of calcium. Bone meal, which comes from the ground bones of young animals, contains calcium from microcrystalline hydroxyapatite. Bone meal calcium is well absorbed, but it is possible for it to be contaminated with heavy metals such as lead. Calcium carbonate, which contains 40 percent elemental calcium, is the most concentrated and cheapest form, but its absorption varies. Calcium lactate, calcium citrate, and calcium gluconate are less concentrated forms of calcium (containing around 15 percent elemental calcium) but are better absorbed than the carbonate forms.

Some calcium supplements contain a mixture of different types of calcium to improve absorption. Many good calcium supplements also contain vitamin D (cholecalciferol), which enhances the absorption of calcium from the intestines. Calcium is best absorbed when taken on an empty stomach, although if need be it can be taken with food. It should not, however, be taken with high-fiber foods such as cereals, grains, and legumes, as this will reduce its absorption. It can be taken with dairy products, fruits, vegetables, or meats.

To test the absorbability of a calcium supplement, place it in vinegar at room temperature for half an hour, stirring it every few minutes. After this time, the supplement should be completely dissolved. If it isn't, then it won't dissolve in your stomach, either, and you should switch to another brand that passes the vinegar test.

Our bones contain magnesium and the trace minerals zinc, silica, boron, and manganese in addition to calcium, and studies suggest that adequate amounts of all these different minerals (see pages 104-107) are more effective than calcium alone at preventing bone loss. If your diet is not always perfect, I suggest that you take a trace mineral tablet that contains all of these minerals. Calcium and other mineral tablets are best taken last thing at night before going to bed.

In addition to making sure you obtain sufficient calcium and other minerals in your diet, avoid making dietary mistakes that can steal minerals from your bones. Keep your consumption of protein from animal sources (meat, fish, dairy products) to no more than 50 grams daily. This is the equivalent of the amount of protein found in a six-ounce serving of meat or fish plus one eight-ounce glass of milk

Food Sources of Calcium

Many different foods contain calcium, but some contain more than others. This table will give you an idea of which foods are the best sources of calcium. Use it to see whether your normal diet is providing you with the recommended 1,000 milligrams of calcium per day. If not, you should either include more calcium-rich foods in your diet or take supplemental calcium to make sure you get enough of this vital mineral.

Avoid foods that contain phosphorus or phosphate additives. These include many processed foods and fizzy soft drinks. If you consume beverages containing alcohol or caffeine, either eliminate these items from your diet or keep your consumption to a moderate or low level.

As a doctor who has treated menopausal women for twenty years, I have seen my attitudes change and evolve over time. In my early days, I believed that hormone replacement therapy was the crucial factor in helping women to cope with menopausal problems and improve their health. In later years, I came to see the vital importance of nutrition and natural medicine. By using specific nutritional supplements and reducing the amount of fat, salt, refined sugars, and chemical additives in your diet, you provide a much stronger foundation for long-lasting health, youthfulness, and vitality than HRT alone could ever provide. The re-energizing power of nutritional and herbal medicine will never cease to amaze you.

Acne

Acne is an inflammatory disorder of the sebaceous (oil) glands located under the skin. When for some reason glandular activity increases, for example puberty, the glands secrete a lot more sebum then normal. If on its way to the surface, the sebum becomes trapped under the skin, the gland breaks, spilling sebum. This irritates the under layers of the skin and some pimples forms. This is how acne begins to affect several body parts, like the face, back, neck or chest.

Oil gets to the surface by traveling up the hair shaft. When the pores become clogged with excess oil and dead cells, the opening narrows; this shuts off oxygen to the pores and encourages bacterial growth, infection and inflammation. Blackheads arise when trapped oil darkens as it oxidizes (although many people mistakenly believe that this darkening of the pore is cause by dirt). When pores are repeatedly clogged, they enlarge and change the skin's texture.

Acne, although common among teenagers, can occur at any time in life and can be caused by allergies, high sugar or diets high in fat. In women Acne can be developed from the use of contraceptives which cause hormone changes. Some drugs such as cortisone or anti epileptics can cause acne as well. In severe cases, it scars and pits the skin.

TIP: Some doctors prescribe a contraceptive pill for girls suffering of acne. This pill contains a hormone called estrogen. The drug suppresses the hormonal actions and produces some dangerous side effects: nausea, vomiting, headaches, weight gain and liver malfunctions.

Acne has become the most treated skin condition in the past few years due to the mental anguish and the impact to the person's self esteem. People who have had acne for a long time report feelings of being unattractive and are very self-conscious about their skin problem. Acne can cause many psychological effects such as low self-esteem, confusion and frustration, anger, depression and social withdrawal.

People suffering from acne often seek help from a dermatologist who almost immediately prescribes antibiotics which can cause terrible side effects, for example, Clindamycin can cause colitis which in turn causes among others bloody stools and in some cases can be fatal. The only drug proven to work in 90% of cases is Isotretinoin, however, it can cause severe side effects, such as nose bleed, dry skin, headaches, joint and muscle pains and the most dangerous, birth defects.

DID YOU KNOW that Tetracycline can permanently stain teeth of unborn children?

The skin is the largest organ in the body. It is in charge of several jobs. One of them is to get rid of some toxins and waste through sweating. If the liver and kidneys can't handle the amount of toxins, then the skin takes over and begins discharging the extra waste. This can have an effect on the skin's health and can cause acne and other disorders.

We recommend

• Colloidal silver is used as a natural antibiotic. Take orally and apply directly on the affected area.

• Take garlic capsules. They boost the immune system and kill the bacteria found in acne.

• To help the liver eliminate toxins from the blood, take Burdock root and dandelion which contain inulin. This helps kill bacteria thus improving the skin.

• Take the homeopathic remedies Kali bromatum, Sulphur, Antimonium tartaricum and Herpa sulphuris. These help prevent the formation of pimples or quickly bring them to a head.

• Use Lavender oil and apply directly on the acne area.

• Put Tea tree oil on the acne affected skin.   This is a natural antibiotic. It will destroy a broad range of invading microorganisms as effectively as benzol peroxide but without side effects. It reduces redness, itchiness and stinging.

• Eat foods high in fiber. This will keep the colon clean.

• Eat Shellfish, soybeans, sunflower seeds and nuts. These are all rich in zinc which is an antibacterial.

- Do not drink alcohol, soft drinks or caffeine. Do not eat eggs, chocolate, fried food, or fats.

- Anything containing sugar can produce what is called "skin diabetes" which leads to acne.

- Drinking lots of water helps clean the body by carrying out waste.

- Do not use electric shavers. They can scar the skin affected by acne.

- Do not wear oil based makeup. Use water based natural makeup instead.

- Some medical journals in Germany show that the herb called vitex berry reduces hormone levels and controls their actions.

- Remember that stress can also cause acne especially in adults. Try to control or avoid stress. Many studies have shown a reduction of acne in people using relaxation techniques.

• Mix chamomile, licorice, elder flowers and red clover   to unclog pores and refine, soften and heal the skin.

Pimple remover solution.

½ cup of boiling water.

2 tsp. Epson salts.

6 drops of lavender essential oil.

Mix water and salts, once the salt is dissolved. Add lavender and soak a cotton cloth and compress on affected area. If cloth cools, soak it again and repeat several times.

Acne Killer (intensive care).

1 tsp. of goldenseal root (powdered).

30 drops of tea tree oil essential oil.

Mix ingredients and form a paste. Apply directly on the acne affected skin and let it dry for 20 minutes. Rinse with lukewarm water.

- If pimples are red and bleeding use calendula. This antiseptic herb prevents scarring, speeds healing and it reduces inflammation.

- Yellow dock can be used as a compress to extract pus from pimples and quickly cure infection.

- Oregon grape is an excellent herb for chronic acne. It prevents pitting scars.

- Red clover is safe for children and very potent. It's used in traditional skin cancer formulas. It's very good for acne on the nose, forehead and scalp. It helps control oily skin.

Acne Healing Juices to be used during a fast.

Fasting helps eliminate toxins from the body especially from the liver and kidneys; this method of cleansing reduces the workload of these organs which in turn work more efficiently, cleaner blood means that fewer impurities are excreted though the skin, thus reducing acne. Try the juices below during fasting as a complementary treatment to the home remedies for acne.

Juices and smoothies

Apple, celery and cucumber juice

Ingredients:

8 apples

1/2 cucumber

6 sticks celery

Directions: Juice all the ingredients. Pour into glasses. Makes approximately 1 pint.

Carrot and mango juice

Ingredients:

8 medium size carrots, peeled or scrubbed

2 large ripe mangoes, peeled and stoned

Directions: Juice the carrots, followed by the mango. Pour into glasses. Makes approximately 1 pint.

Carrot, apple and ginger juice

Ingredients:

8 apples, washed and chopped but not peeled

4 carrots, peeled or scrubbed

1 inch ginger root, peeled

Directions: Juice the apples, then the carrots and finally the ginger. Pour into glasses.

Makes approximately 1 pint.

Alzheimer's disease

Alzheimer's disease is a common type of dementia, or decline in intellectual function.

Once thought rare, Alzheimer's disease is now known to affect more than 4.1 million people in the United States. It afflicts 10 percent of Americans over 65 years of age and as many as 50 percent of those over 85 years old. However, the disease does not affect only the elderly, but may strike when a person is in his or her forties. Most people over forty are using some type of alternative or home remedies to prevent the early development of Alzheimer's disease.

What is Alzheimer's disease?

This disorder was first identified in 1906 by a German neurologist named Alois

Alzheimer. It is characterized by progressive mental deterioration to such a degree that it interferes with one's ability to function socially and at work. Memory and abstract thoughts process are affected. Alzheimer's disease is irreversible and progressive disorder that since 1906 very little progress has been made by conventional medicine to slow or prevent it. However, there are many home remedies for Alzheimer's disease that have shown remarkable results in preventing and in some cases restore mental deterioration.

I have very pour memory. Do I have Alzheimer's disease?

Many people worry that their forgetfulness is a sign of Alzheimer's disease. The fact is that most of us forget where we put our car keys or our glasses or someone's birthday but this is not a sign of Alzheimer's disease. A few good example of the difference between forgetfulness and Alzheimer's is the following: If you forget where you put your car keys that is forgetfulness, if you do not remember whether or not you have a car, that is Alzheimer's, or if you forget where you put your glasses that is forgetfulness, if you do not remember whether or not you use glasses that is Alzheimer's. Forgetfulness is also very frustrating and can also be improved by using some very powerful home remedies for memory loss.

What causes Alzheimer's disease?

The precise cause or causes of Alzheimer's are unknown, but research reveals a number of interesting clues. Many of them point to nutritional deficiencies. For example, people with Alzheimer's tend to have low levels of vitamin B12 and zinc in their bodies. The B vitamins are important in cognitive functioning, and well known that processed foods have been stripped from this nutrients. In addition the average sixty year old person is likely to be taking between 8 and 10 prescription and over-the-counter drugs, these potential drug reactions and pour diet often interfere or adversely affect mentally and physically since many medications deplete crucial vitamins and minerals.

Low levels of antioxidants vitamin A and E and carotenoids are also present in people suffering from Alzheimer's. These nutrients act as free radicals scavengers; damage caused by free radicals may expose the brain cells to increased oxidative damage.

How can I treat Alzheimer's naturally with home remedies?

• According to a report published in the October 22, 1977 edition of the Journal of the American Medical Association (JAMA), Ginkgo biloba extract can stabilize and in some cases improve the mental functioning and social behavior of people with Alzheimer's disease. Take 100 to 200 mg of ginkgo biloba extract 3 times a day.

• The Chinese herb Qian Ceng to (Huperzia serata) increases memory retention. This is the same herb that is the source of huperzine A, and it is also known as club moss.

Pure and standardized extracts of this herb have been shown to increase clear-headedness, language ability and memory retention in a significantly high percentage of subjects with Alzheimer's disease. It is a potent blocker of acetylcholinesterase, an enzyme that regulates the activity of acetylcholine, which is an important chemical of the brain that maintains healthy learning and memory functions.

• Valerian root improves sleep patterns when taken as bedtime.

• Eat a well-balanced diet of natural foods and follow the supplementation program mention above.

• Folate and Vitamin B12 prevent elevated levels of homocysteine, a chemical that increases the risk for Alzheimer's disease and heart disease. This vitamin may be important for preventing or delaying the symptoms of Alzheimer's disease. This vitamin is added to cereal products Foods containing folate include avocados, bananas, oranges, asparagus, green leafy vegetables, and dried beans. B12 is found only in animal products. (Oily fish are very high in B12 and also have other nerve-protective properties.). I recommend 400 mcg of folic acid to reduce homocysteine, although one study suggested 800 mcg (.8 mg) a day is necessary to reduce homocysteine levels.

• Avoid alcohol, cigarette smoke, processed foods, and metal pollutants like aluminum, and mercury.

TIP: Did you know that in a study published in the British Medical Journal, smoking doubles the chances of developing dementia and Alzheimer's?

• The herbs balm and sage are being researched for possible beneficial effects and brain chemistry. Balm appears to simulate the neurological receptors that bind acetylcholine. Sage contains compounds that are cholinesterase inhibitors.

• Vitamin E can slow the progression of Alzheimer's disease by as much as 25% according to a study in 1997.

• A study conducted by the research department at Oakwood college in Alabama sowed that liquid aged garlic extract (kyolic) may be useful in the improvement of Alzheimer's disease symptoms.

Anemia:

Anemia is a decrease in your blood cell count and/or a decreased hemoglobin content in the blood. Since red blood cells are the ones responsible for carrying oxygen to the cells via the hemoglobin, a lower amount would mean low oxygen in all your body's tissues and your baby would get less oxygen as well. Anemia can be caused by blood loss which means that not enough red cells are being produced or that too many red cells are being killed off. During pregnancy, the blood volume in your baby increases by about 40%.

Most women during their pregnancy become anemic because their bodies are not producing enough red cells and it is usually caused by a nutritional deficiency. Late in the second trimester, the hematocrit decreases but this does not make you anemic. Hematocrit is the percentage of red blood cell volume of the total blood volume.

Usually anemia is due to iron deficiency but also can be caused by not having enough Vitamin B12; B6; Folic acid, and/or copper in your system. During your pregnancy blood counts will be done that will help to determine what vitamins or nutrients you are lacking but in some cases more specific tests are needed. These might include blood work for Iron; Vitamin B12; Ferritin; Iron binding capacity and folic acid level. Just taking Iron is not always the answer. That's why it's important to find out the real cause of Anemia from blood test. Anemia has the following symptoms:

•You feel fatigued.

•You feel dizzy.

•You lack vitality.

•You are short of breath.

•Your skin looks white as well as your gums and around your eyes.

If you have Anemia at the time of delivery you will be at risk of losing excessive blood and going into shock. Your baby also may have low amounts of Iron stored for the first month of life.

TIP: There is another type of Anemia called "Pica." In this kind of Anemia you may have rare cravings, for example you will want to eat substances other than food, such as, coal, dirt, starch or hair. This kind of Anemia is usually the sign of a nutritional deficiency.

We recommend:

•It's very important to get the proper nutrients into the body. Eat a diet rich in cereals, rice, pastas, dairy products (milk, yogurt and cheese), vegetables and fruits, meat, poultry and fish and finally dry beans, eggs, and nuts. These foods have been proven to help boost the immune system.

•Make sure you are eating plenty of iron rich food such as, liver, green leafy vegetables, beets, dried fruits, bran flakes, oysters, brown rice, lentils and molasses, raisins, prunes; breads and pastas made of whole grain flour.

•Avoid drinking coffee, tea and ingesting antacids, because they decrease iron absorption.

•Try to cook in iron pots; it is proven that doing it can increase significantly the amount of iron in your foods.

•During your pregnancy it's important to take the correct vitamins that will help you and your baby be healthy. Here are the following required during this period:

Vitamin A: 5,000 IU

Vitamin E: 400 IU

Vitamin B1: 1.5 mg

Vitamin K: 65 mg

Vitamin B2: 1.6 mg

Calcium: 1,200 mg

Vitamin B3: 17 mg

Magnesium: 500 mg

Vitamin B6: 2.2 mg

Iron: 30 mg

Vitamin B12: 2.2 mcg

Phosphorous: 1,200 mg

Folic Acid: 800 mcg

Iodine: 175 mcg

Vitamin C: 500-1,000 mg

Selenium: 65 mcg

Vitamin D: 400 IU

•In addition take an organic form of Iron (amino acid chelate): 100 mg of elemental Iron daily (Iron aspararte, citrate or picolinate), not the poorly absorbed sulphate which may cause constipation and/or stomach ache.

•Vitamin C (500 mg) is recommended to be taken with iron for better absorption. Desiccated liver tablets may be helpful as well and a Folic acid supplement with Vitamin B6 and B12 should be used to prevent anemia.

•Also herbs can help your body maintain a good level of iron, such as:

½ to 1 tsp. of the tincture of Yellow dock root three times daily, or
½ to 1 tsp. of extract of Dandelion leaf and/or root or two capsules twice daily, or
Eat Dandelion greens in your salads.

Here are some homeopathic remedies:
•Take China if the cause of the anemia is due to loss of blood or fluids.

•If your skin looks pale or white, shiny or a little green, take

Calcarea Phosphoric.

•If your face looks red and then suddenly turns pale and your feet and hands swell take Foram acet.

•To improve the quality of your red blood cells in your body take Foram Phosphoric which can also be taken with Calcarea Phosphorica.

•If you take Calcarea Phosphorica use a 3X potency that will help you build up your hemoglobin level.

•If your gums look white and your blood rushes to your head when you lay down take Graphite.

•If your body feels cold and chilly or if the cause of your anemia is due to loss of blood because you have menstrual disorders take Natrum Muriaticum.

•If you are not thirsty and your body is cold and you feel tired and your condition improves being outdoors take Pulsatilla.

•Eat alfalfa. This nutritive herb promotes digestion/assimilation of vitamins minerals. An excellent source of nutrients, it's needed for iron absorption and blood clotting including B6, E, K, Iron, potassium, zinc, magnesium.

•Dong Quai is a Chinese herb rich in B12 and folic acid. It treats iron deficiency anemia increases the production of red blood cells and combats weakness and fatigue. It also protects the liver.

•For anemia after or before childbirth use Raspberry leaf. it is very rich in iron and calcium and also helpful for excess loss of blood due to injury or menstruation.

•A very good blood tonic is found in the herb called yellow dock. It assists in the assimilation of dietary iron.

Arthritis

Arthritis is a prehistoric disease; archeologists have found skeletons of the first humans with evident cases of arthritis. But modern medicine has not yet found the reason why this condition affects more than 100 million people around the world.

Arthritis affects the joints of the body. They become swollen, painful, deformed and stiff and eventually the joint loses range of motion and the pain becomes unbearable. There are many types of arthritis; the most common one is Osteoarthritis which causes a slow deterioration of the cartilage on the tip of each bone. The bones then start rubbing against each other injuring the articulation and scar tissue grows to deform the area.

There are several drugs that deal with the pain and inflammation of arthritis but most of them don't do a very good job considering all the side effects they cause. For example ibuprofen (Advil) or naproxen (Aleve) and even other more powerful prescription drugs cause severe gastrointestinal problems such as bleeding ulcers, acidosis and stomach pain. They interfere with the synthesis of collagen which is fundamental for the formation of cartilage. If cartilage is not rebuilding itself more damage is going to be inflicted on the joints.

Although the commercials on television tell us it is safe to take over the counter drugs every day and many people suffering from arthritis do, the truth is that they cause damage to other parts of the body which is a price too high to pay just too high to temporarily get rid of pain and inflammation.

But not everybody knows this. When they start to experience gastrointestinal problems a drug is prescribed to deal with that condition suppressing the stomach acid in order to cure the ulcers in their stomach. This causes incomplete digestion (not enough acid to dissolve food) which leads to an insufficient absorption of nutrients, low level malnutrition, fatigue and depressed immune systems. At this point a person can be taking anywhere from 6 to 10 pills a day, then quality of life starts to go downhill just because they have arthritis pain.

Some people suffering all these side effects opt to take acetaminophen (Tylenol) because it works blocking the nerve impulses to the brain that trigger the pain sensation. This drug will not cause ulcers and gastrointestinal bleeding. The problem is that it does not control inflammation and an inflamed joint with no pain sensation is likely to be severely damaged because you don't feel the pain and you push the joint to perform resulting in grater damage to the whole articulation.

If you are one of the lucky ones who don´t have gastrointestinal problems you still need to be careful bacause these drugs also cause liver and kidney damage when used daily for prolonged periods of time.

There is a drug called celecoxib (Celebrex) this is one big money maker to the drug company, in the first three months in the market it was prescribed to about 2.5 million people in the United States alone. This is a very expensive drug about 2 US$ per pill and still has severe side effects. It's been linked to more then ten deaths, half of them due to gastrointestinal hemorrhage. The FDA has requested that the safety information of all of these products include information about cardiovascular and gastrointestinal risks.

Since there is no cure for arthritis and the risk of damage that could be generated by drugs is great, we suggest that you take a good look at all the natural remedies that have been with us since the year 500 AD. Mother earth gives us some very powerful herbs that can reduce arthritis pain and inflammation and combined with nutrients, mineral and vitamins are sure to get rid of the symptoms of arthritis without side effects and without chemicals.

We recommend

TIP: Any kind of infection anywhere in the body can contribute to causing Arthritis.

• Eat Alfalfa or take alfalfa capsules. It's very rich in minerals needed for the formation of bones.

• Take chondroitin sulfate 700 mg. a day to strengthen joints and ligaments.

• Take Vitamin E to protect and improve joint mobility.

• Bogbean is a very powerful aquatic herb for for rheumatoid arthritis and Osteoarthritis It is anti-inflammatory and cleans the urinary tract so drink lots of water.

• Boswellia has anti-inflammatory effects similar to Non-steroidal anti-inflammatory drugs (NSAID) (Advil, Aleve, Tylenol etc.) but this herb does not have side effects and does not cause gastrointestinal bleeding. It improves circulation to the joints, relieves pain, inflammation and stiffness.

• Ginger is the Killer of Arthritis pain. Superior to any NASID, it can be applied directly on the affected area or taken orally, either way it relieves pain, inflammation, stiffness, bursitis and tendinitis.

• Curcumin stimulates the production of cortisone better or equal to cortisone and anti-inflammatory drugs.   It's an antioxidant and anti-inflammatory especially good for rheumatoid arthritis and Osteoarthritis. Take it orally or externally.

• Cayennes is very helpful for pain. Use it as an external ointment. It improves circulation.

• Bromelain comes from the stem of the pineapple and contains anti-inflammatory blocks, reduces swelling, pain and damage to joints. A study done on 200 people showed a 75% reduction in inflammation which is better than that obtained using drugs. In the last few years Bromelain has been used in hospitals across U.S.

Arthritis pain relief remedy.

Mix 2 tsp. of devil's claw tuber.

2 tsp. of white willow bark.

1 tsp. feverfew.

2 tsp. yucca root.

2 tsp. sarsaparilla root.

3 cups of water.

Soak all ingredients in the water for eight hours, drain and drink 1/2 a cup 3 times a day.

• Du Huo Gashing is a Chinese herbal medicine that has proven to be helpful for arthritis.

• Nettle leaf is used in Germany for arthritis.

• A combination of ash bark, aspen bark and goldenrod has been used in Germany for 30 years to treat arthritis.

• Eating 20 cherries a day is more effective than Aspirin in relieving pain and inflammation.

TIP: Women with silicone breast implants are at a very high risk of developing antibodies that can attack collagen causing damage to joints, tendons and ligaments.

• To repair and rebuild bones and cartilage, eat foods rich in sulfur such as eggs, garlic and onion.

• Eat fresh pineapple. As mention before it contains Bromelain, an anti-inflammatory enzyme.

• Vitamin D3 is needed for good bone formation. Remember that the sun gives it for free. Spend time outdoors in order to get sunshine because it promotes the synthesis of vitamin D3.

• Soak a cotton rag in hot castor oil wrap the affected area with the cloth, place a piece of plastic over it and apply a heating pad to keep the oil warm. This is very helpful in relieving stiffness and pain.

• Combining the Chinese herbs blupleurum, ginseng and licorice will be very helpful in reducing or completely relieving pain resulting from inflammation. These herbs reverse the damage caused by the drug Prednisone which is used for the same condition but the herbs produce no side effects.

• The herb Cat's Claw grows in South America has been researched and proven to reduce inflammation while boosting the immune system. These studies also discovered that cat's claw contains anti-arthritic compounds and is currently being used to treat people with rheumatoid arthritis.

• Injections made with the herb Devil's claw are prescribed by physicians in Europe. It's also used in ointment and tea to reduce arthritis pain and inflammation.

Inflammation and pain Tincture.

1/2 tsp. of bupleurum root tincture.

1/2 tsp. of ginseng root tincture.

1/2 tsp. of licorice root tincture.

1/2 tsp. of echinacea root tincture.

1/2 tsp. of yucca root tincture.

Combine all ingredients and take half a dropperful three times a day.

Asthma

TIP: Medication used to treat high blood pressure can cause life threatening complications in people with asthma.

Asthma is a very common respiratory disease.   It affects the trachea and bronchial tubes which become inflamed and plugged with mucus. This causes the airways to narrow restricting the amount of air going to the lungs and makes it very difficult to breathe. Asthma can occur in anyone but is very common in children and early adulthood. Typical symptoms of an asthma attack are coughing, wheezing, tight chest and difficulty breathing.

There are two types of asthma: allergic and non allergic. Some of the allergens that can trigger an asthma attack are chemicals, drugs, smoke, dust, food additives, pollution, mold, etc. Non allergic asthma can be caused by anxiety, exercise, dry or humid weather, fear, laughing, stress etc.

The rate in which asthma attacks has increased in the past few years is alarming, especially in children. Scientists believe that there is a strong link between contamination in the air we breathe and asthma. Evidence suggests that the percentage of people who live in big cities and have asthma attacks is far greater than those of people who live in rural areas. However this may not be the only reason. Genetics food additives, toxins etc also play a part.

Modern medicine can offer very little to children with asthma. Most drugs can only produce a temporary effect. Herbs on the other hand can be very helpful not only reducing attacks but also strengthening the lungs and immune system. You'll learn to treat this disease with many combinations of herbs such as mullein, elecampane and more.

TIP: Did you know that aspirin, Advil, chemotherapy and antibiotics can cause asthma attacks?

We recommend

- Vitamin B6 and Vitamin B12.They are very important nutrients to treat asthma by decreasing the inflammation in the lungs.

- Vitamin C Is needed to fight infection, increase the amount of oxygen and reduce inflammation.

- Use ginkgo biloba. This herb contains ginkgolide B which is very helpful. Some studies indicate that ginkgo biloba reduces the frequency of asthma attacks.

- Mullein oil is used to fight respiratory congestion. It is very important to make it as a tea for faster results.

- Pau d'arco is a natural antibiotic and reduces inflammation.

• In China a powerful mixture of herbs called Shuan Huang Lian is being used in hospitals to treat respiratory illness. It is very important to use this herb to treat asthma and acute bronchitis.

• If exercise triggers asthma attacks, cut back the amount of salt in your diet and take 2,000 mg. of Vitamin C one hour before your workout.

• Eat salmon 3 times a week and take salmon oil capsules.

• Drink coffee and soft drinks with caffeine (colas). Caffeine dilates the bronchial airways.

Make a tea using:

2 tsp. powdered Indian root.

2 tsp. granulated echinacea root.

2 tsp. elecampane root.

2 cups of water.

Mix all ingredients and let them set for 2 hours.

To improve breathing make a tea with:

1 quart boiling water.

1 tsp. chamomile flowers.

1 tsp. echinacea root.

1 tsp. mullein leaves.

1 tsp. passionflower leaves.

Mix herbs and pour boiling water over them, steep for 20 minutes, strain and give ½ a cup a day.

Throat spray for asthma attacks. (This remedy is used as many asthmatic inhalers).

1 tsp. ginkgo leaves (tincture form).

5 drops chamomile essential oil.

1/4 cup of water.

Mix all the liquids and store them in a spray or pump bottle to use as needed. This remedy keeps airways clear and dilated.

• A very tasteful herb for children is Lemon verbena tea. This herb reduces wheezing and doctors recommend it in South America.

• If you have a baby make sure you breast feed. This has been shown to greatly improve the chances of not getting asthma in the first place.

Chinese preparation remedy.

1 tsp. magnolia flowers.

1 tsp. rehmannia root.

½ tsp. don quai root.

3 cups of water.

Boil all ingredients and simmer for 15 minutes, remove from heat and steep for another 15 minutes, strain and give one cup a day.

• In recent studies scientists in Germany discovered that onion contains some compounds that are very helpful with asthma. Drink one glass of onion juice a day. If your child will not drink onion juice you can try to add onion to his or her food.

• Jamaican dogwood is a strong pain reliever, sedative and antispasmodic. It's very helpful for muscular back pain, asthma, menstrual pain, insomnia, toothaches, and nervous conditions.

Back Pain:

About 80% of adults suffer from back pain at some time in their lives. Backaches are categorized as acute and chronic. Acute pain is caused by movement or excessive use of the back which can injure the muscles, ligaments, bones, tendons.

Chronic pain is a recurring backache that restricts of normal movements for no particular reason and can also affect the tendons, ligaments and bones.

Problems with some organs can cause back pain as well, for example, kidney infection, prostate problems, female pelvic disorder, bladder and even constipation can be felt in the lower back.

Back pain is very common during pregnancy due to the considerable anatomical changes and stress in the body. Carrying a child changes the position of your internal organs putting a huge amount of pressure on the lower spine. The increase in body weight, the muscle relaxing effects of the hormone progesterone and the change in your center of gravity contribute to the problem. That's why every day as your baby grows it's harder to get up and down from chairs and beds.

If you have back pain you can also feel muscle aches, locked areas in your back, stiff neck and your whole body will ache.

Other causes of back pain can be poor postural habits, strains, microtrauma, muscle tension and nutritional deficiencies. When repeated episodes of injury are added to this mix, the discs become thin, deteriorated or ruptured. These events can also lead to arthritic related conditions. With nerves close by, swelling or compression in the spine often results in neuritis, lumbar neuralgia, or sciatica.

Herbal medicines are used in these conditions with far more safety then drugs especially in pregnant women.

We recommend

•Ask someone to massage the affected area with herbal oils using knuckles and increasing pressure slowly. After a few minutes you will feel less discomfort. This gets rid of tension and relaxes the muscles in that area.

•Every time you lift something, remember to bend your knees first. This will prevent your lower back from getting tense and causing damage to your spine and back muscles.

•Never twist while lifting as this can have a bad effect on your vertebrates.

•Avoid lifting heavy objects in the last couple of weeks of your pregnancy.

•Do not sit in couches. Always sit in firm chairs supporting the lumbar area with a pillow. This will help you keep your waist and lower back in the proper position.

•Apply St. john's Wort directly to the back area. CAUTION: Do not suntan as this oil makes your skin very sensitive to the sun.

•Do not wear high heel shoes. They change your center of gravity even more, increasing the risk of falling and they put more pressure on your back. Instead wear well fitted, well-padded flat shoes that support your feet and provide ample room for your toes.

•Try to sleep with pillows supporting your back, legs and belly.

•Here are some homeopathic remedies that will help you with back pains, Cimicifuga, Kali carbonica. Lincopodium, Nux vomica and Arnica.

•Black Haw contains compounds very similar to the ones found in aspirin. It relieves spasms and neuralgia of back and neck, sciatica, leg cramps, tension headaches and wry neck.

•Boswellia is a strong anti-inflammatory which reduces stiffness and pain. It has to be used for at least 4 weeks in chronic cases. It improves circulation around ligaments, joints and tendons.

•Jamaican dogwood is a strong pain reliever, sedative and antispasmodic. It's very helpful for muscular back pain, asthma, menstrual pain, insomnia, toothaches, and nervous conditions.

•Dong quai has 1.5 times the analgesic activity of aspirin. It relieves back pain, cramping, muscular spasms and inflammation.

•The herb Cat's claw grows in South America has been researched and proven to reduce inflammation while boosting the immune system. The studies also discovered that cat's claw contains anti arthritic compounds and is currently being used to treat people with rheumatoid arthritis.

•Take Vitamin E to protect and improve joint mobility.

•Bromelain comes from the stem of the pineapple. It contains anti-inflammatory blocks, reduces swelling, pain and damage to joints. A study done on 200 people showed a 75% greater reduction in inflammation than the ones obtained using drugs. Finally in the last few years bromelain is being used in hospitals across U.S.

•Wild yam, is used for back pain characterized by sharp, knifelike sensations.

•Barberry is used for low back pain often related to kidney weakness. Good also for sciatica and neuralgia with radiating pain.

•Horsetail has high amounts of silica which is essential for bones and connective tissue.

•Eat alfalfa or take alfalfa extract in capsules. It contains all the necessary nutrients to alleviate back pain.

TIP: A homemade ice pack can be made by mixing 2 parts water and 1 part alcohol in a nylon bag and freezing it. The bag will be flexible thus molding to the body and it will not sweat.

•When pain hits suddenly, drink two large glasses of pure water. Dehydration can cause back pain.

•Several studies done in Scandinavia on smoking and non smoking twins have shown that smoking greatly aggravates problems in the disks. It's always advisable to quit smoking.

•Rhus toxicodendrom is a homeopathic remedy that relieves stiffness.

High Cholesterol:

There are two types of cholesterol: Low density lipoproteins or LDL (bad cholesterol) and High density lipoproteins HDL (good cholesterol). LDLs are responsible for plaque buildup in the arteries which block the flow of blood to major organs like the liver, the kidneys, genitals and brain and is the number one cause of heart disease.

HDLs in the other hand are considered good because they carry unused cholesterol back to the liver where it was produced. Once there the liver breakes it down to be removed from the body. The needed cholesterol plays an important part in the formation of sex hormones and proper nerve and brain function. However if we do not have enough HDLs or too much cholesterol for them to pick up and transport back to the liver it will stay in our arteries blocking them.

But you are probably asking yourself if the cholesterol is produced in the liver,   why would I have too much? It seems like the liver would regulate how much cholesterol is needed. That is right. The problem is that cholesterol is also present in our diet and usually we eat too much saturated fats such as coconuts, white bread, gravies, pork products, etc. and all these added to the cholesterol produced by the liver could make us reach an unsafe cholesterol level.

The number considered to be safe for both LDL and HDL is 200 mg./dl (milligrams per deciliter). A reading above 200 is a sign of potential development of heart disease, a level of 240 is considered to be at high risk. It is also important to maintain a good level of HDLs, 80 mg./dl. is recommended. A reading of 35 HDL would be considered very low even if the total level is below 200 mg./dl.

There are drugs to keep LDL levels low but these drugs can cause side effects including vomiting, headaches, impotence, internal bleeding and vitamin deficiencies including Coenzyme Q10, the heart's most important nutrient. Why experience all that when there is a better way to keep cholesterol levels at an acceptable number. Taking herbs, vitamins and cutting fats from our diet is the safest way of ensuring a low risk of developing heart disease.

We recommend

Mix 1 tsp. of roasted chicory root.

1 tsp. of lime flowers.

½ tsp. of fenugreek seeds.

½ tsp. of ginger rhizome.

1 quart of water.

Boil all ingredients, let cool, strain. Drink 2 cups a day.

• Eat Garlic or take 1 capsule twice a day. It lowers LDL cholesterol level by 12% and increases HDLs.

• Take 400 mcg. a day of chromium picolinate to improve HDL to LDL ratio.

• Taking 4000 mg. Vitamin C with bioflavonoids a day lowers cholesterol.

• Ginger reduces cholesterol and thins the blood improving circulation.

• Guggul reduces LDL by 35% and increases HDL by 20 % in 12 weeks to prevent arteriosclerosis. It has performed better then many drugs in several studies.

• Red Rice Yeast is a Chinese medicine that lowers cholesterol, improves circulation and strengthens the heart.

• Eat vegetables and fruits as they are cholesterol free.

• Spirulina taken daily has been shown to lower cholesterol.

• Olive oil, bananas, apples, carrots, dried beans, garlic and grapefruit are the cholesterol lowering foods.

• Studies have shown that almonds lower cholesterol by 16 points in four weeks.

• Meat and dairy products are the number one source of cholesterol.

COLDS:

There are more than 150 viruses that can cause colds. These viruses infect the upper respiratory tract and they thrive in cold temperature so it is very common to catch a cold during fall or winter. Sometimes colds are mistaken for Flu but there are very distinct differences between the two. Flu is a lot more severe with fever that ranges from 102 to 104 F. While colds very rarely develop a fever. Colds last for about a week or so but if treated in the early stages can be reduced to a few days.

In the United States $1 billion a year is wasted on nonprescription drugs for colds and coughs but often these medicines do not help the cold itself but the symptoms which are necessary tools for the body to heal itself. An example would be taking an analgesic for pain and fever such as Aspirin or Ibuprofen. Colds develop very little if any fever, a higher fever may be indication of a more serious problem. Taking these products can mask this condition. When our nose runs it is because the body is creating mucus, a secretion that traps the virus and expels it from the body. By taking an antihistamine we decrease this secretion thus keeping the virus inside. Natural remedies help the immune system fight the virus, vitamins help boost our defenses and herbs help reduce pain etc.

We recommend: At the first sign of a cold:

• Take Vitamin C and Zinc lozenges. This can help stop the cold from going through the entire process.

• Take Echinacea and goldenseal extracts. These boost the immune system.

• Put eucalyptus oil in 2 cups of boiling water and breath in the steam to help with congestion.

• Native Americans use Hyssop in tea form as an expectorant and to fight viruses.

• Gargle: A mix of water and pure tea tree oil helps sore throats.

• Drink chicken broth and potato peeling broth.

• Do not use handkerchiefs. Use paper tissues and flush them after use. The cold virus lives for several hours thus increasing the risk of reinfecting yourself.

• Wash your hands frequently to reduce the chances of re infecting yourself and others.

• Other homeopathic remedies are: Belladonna; Arsenicum; Aconite and Antimonium tartaricum.

• Take echinacea. This herb is antiviral and antibacterial, speeds healing and boosts the immune system.

• Horseradish is another herb that many use in the kitchen but also has excellent properties to treat sore throat and upper respiratory tract infections. It reduces fever and expels concentrations of mucus.

• Use kava kava as a gargle for soothing and analgesic pain relief. Helps insomnia caused by coughing and sore throat.

• Myrrh is an antiseptic and anti-inflammatory. it is very powerful and excellent for chronic sore throats. It also acts as an expectorant and decongestant and it helps cure gum disease.

• In Europe it is common to see singers use oregano oil to fight respiratory allergies, laryngitis and sore throat for it's antifungal and antibacterial properties.

• Sage is used to cure sore throat, stuffed nose, gingivitis and coughs. It is a powerful antiviral, antibacterial and antifungal. Use as a gargle.

• Wild indigo is an antiviral and antibiotic for infections. It stimulates the immune system and cures chronic sore throats.

• Mullein coats the throat with a mucus like film helping reduce the burning feeling. It clears mucus and phlegm.

• Osha is an antiviral that works great in the first stages of an infection, colds and flu, sore throat or phlegm and acts as an expectorant.

• Poke root relieves inflammation and infection and reduces coughing, pain and burning.

Make a gargle tonic with:

1 cup of boiling water.

2 tsp. sage leaves.

salt.

Mix all ingredients and let them steep for 30 minutes, drain and use as gargle when needed.

Make your own cough syrup mixing:

1 tbs. licorice root.

1 tbs. of marshmallow root.

1 tbs. of plantain leaves.

1 tsp. of thyme leaf.

4 tbs. of honey.

4 ounces of glycerin.

2 drops of anise oil.

Place all herbs in a container with boiling water, let it simmer for 20 minutes, strain, add honey, glycerin, and if desired, anise. Take one tbs. as needed. Keep in the refrigerator for several months.

Caution:Do not give honey to a child less than 2 years of age. It can be very harmful to them.

Cold and Flu tea.

½ tsp. echinacea root.

½ tsp. peppermint leaves.

½ tsp. hyssop leaves.

½ tsp. yarrow leaves.

½ tsp. elder flowers.

½ tsp. shizandra berries.

1 quart of boiling water.

Mix all ingredients and simmer for 30 minutes, strain and drink several cups a day.

Famous Cold remedy.

30 drops yarrow tincture.　　•Do not• use if pregnant.

60 drops elderberry tincture.

20 drops peppermint leaves tincture.

4 cups of boiling water.

Add tinctures to water let it cool and drink 3 tablespoons every 4 hours.

Constipation:

Constipation refers to any irregularity in, or absence of, bowel movements. The slow movement of food through the large intestine and the amount of time the waste remains in the colon are factors that contribute to constipation. More and more water is absorbed while the waste is in our body and the stool becomes drier and bulky thus more difficult to pass.

Regular bowel movement is necessary to remove waste and toxins from the body. Some people will have movements every day; others three times a week. This is normal although some doctors consider a person moving bowels less than once a day to be constipated.

TIP: It was once believed that castor oil was a good remedy for constipation but we know now that it can cause dehydration and mineral imbalance.

Constipation can be caused by lack of exercise, too much junk food, poor diet, painkillers, antidepressants and/or pregnancy. However, serious diseases can cause constipation as well, including thyroid problems, circulatory disorder, diverticulitis, colon malfunction (fistulas, polyps, tumors, and obstruction).

TIP: Some drugs like cough syrups, codeine, blood pressure medication, calcium supplements and antihistamines can cause constipation.

In pregnant women constipation is normal due to the enlargement of the uterus pressing on the lower intestine. It is very important to improve bowel movement while pregnant since the body is getting rid of waste and toxins coming from two persons. Do not take laxatives because they can cross the placenta barrier and cause untold damage to the baby.

Sometimes constipation can be relieved by a change in diet. Usually, people who don't eat sufficient fibers (fruits and vegetables) and don't drink enough fluids suffer from constipation.

Herbs can relieve constipation but they should be used with care. Herbal laxatives take several hours to start working, between 6 and 24 hours to be exact. If you take too much eventually the laxative will work and since too much was taken diarrhea will develop.

The following instruction will get rid of constipation. We'll teach you how to make a laxative syrup, extra strength laxatives for severe constipation and some potent herbal teas. Take any combination of the remedies in the recommended doses.

We recommend

• Take Apple pectin. It helps with constipation and brings fibers into the body.

• Take folic acid. An insufficient intake of folic acid can lead to constipation.

• To clean and heal the digestive system take, Aloe Vera juice twice a day.

- Ginger tea helps start bowel movement.

- Yerba mate in tea form is very helpful with constipation.

- Eat lots of fruits, green vegetables, cabbage, peas, carrots, garlic and sweet potatoes. All these are high in fiber.

- Exercise. Often a simple stroll in the park can relieve constipation.

- Do not take Epson salts and magnesia. Because they force the body to get rid of essential minerals.

Make a tea mixing the following:

10 boneset flowers.

10 dandelion flowers.

4 ounces of cascara bark.

2 liters of water.

Boil until reduced to half it's initial volume, add 2 tsp. of honey. Drink

2 cups a day.

Constipation relief formula.

2 tsp. cascara sagrada.

2 slices of ginger.

1 tsp. cayenne.

1 tsp. oregon grape root.

Add boiling water, let it sit for one hour. Drink 2 cups a day.

• Drink lots of water (8 glasses a day). it helps to soften stools.

• Eat prunes and drink prune juice. This is one of the best ways to relieve constipation. They act as natural laxatives. Prune juice may be the most effective and gentlest remedy for constipation.

• Cascara also known as cascara sagrada stimulates normal intestinal contractions by increasing water and salts in the bowels which tones the intestinal muscle.

• Chinese rhubarb is a stimulating laxative and purgative with astringent, cleansing effects. It does not cause excessive cramping but removes toxic bacteria from intestines and improves appetite.

• For occasional constipation use Flaxseed (also known as linseed), psyllium, or fenugreek. These herbs are concidered bulk laxatives. Flaxseed has no side effects. You can take one tablespoon of whole seeds two to three times a day followed by two cups of liquid. Drinking lots of fluid during the day is essential for these remedies to work properly.

• Dandelion root is a mild laxative good for chronic constipation. Take one tsp. of Dandelion root boiled in water three or four times a day.

Extra strength fruit and herb laxative.

½ tsp. licorice root.

½ cup of water.

3 stewed prunes.

Bring licorice root and water to a boil and simmer for 5 minutes.
Remove from heat and steep for 5 minutes. Strain and add fruits, let
them soak for 2 hours, eat them warm or cold as needed.

Natural laxative syrup.

1 tsp. honey.

2 tsp. cascara sagrada bark tincture.

1 tsp. licorice root tincture.

½ tsp. fennel tincture.

½ tsp. peppermint tincture.

Warm honey to liquefy it then add tinctures. Stir well and take 2 tsp.
a day.

Dandruff

Dandruff occurs when skin cells renew themselves and the old cells are shed, producing irritating white flakes. Some people tend to generate and discard skin cells at a faster rate than others. Dandruff can be caused by trauma, illness, hormonal disorders, improper diet (specially the consumption of carbohydrates and sugar), deficiency of nutrients such as, B- Complex Vitamins, essential fatty acids, and selenium. Dandruff is worse during the winter. There is no cure for Dandruff, but you can minimize the condition with some powerful Natural remedies.

As we all know, it is an embarrassing problem because it is very noticeable and very itchy and sore if we do not treat it rapidly.

We recommend:

•Use flaxseed oil, primrose oil or salmon oil. They help relieve itching and inflammation. They also promote healthy skin and scalp.

•Take kelp. It improves hair growth and heals the scalp.

•Take Vitamin B complex + extra Vitamin B6 and Vitamin B12. All the B vitamins are needed to obtain a healthy skin and hair.

•Take Selenium. It is an antioxidant which aids in controlling a dry scalp.

•Take Vitamin E. It improves blood circulation.

•Take Vitamin A. It helps prevent dry skin and promote the healing of tissue.

•Take Vitamin C + Bioflavonoids. It is an important antioxidant which prevents tissue damage to the scalp and is a good healing nutrient.

•To rinse your hair use an infusion of Chaparral or Thyme. They are gentle to your hair.

Herbal conditioner for dandruff.

1 pint of water.

1 tsp. of burdock root.

1 tsp. of calendula flowers.

1 tsp. of chamomile flowers.

1 tsp. of lavender flowers.

1 tsp. of rosemary leaves.

1 tbs. of vinegar.

6 drops of sage essential oil.

Boil water and pour over herbs. Steep for 20 minutes strain and add vinegar. Apply after shampooing, do not rinse out.

•Eat a balanced diet including at least 50 to 70% of raw food.

•Avoid dairy products, fried foods, flour, chocolate, nuts, seafood and sugar.

•Make a paste mixing 8 tbs. of pure organic peanut oil and the juice of half a lemon. Before washing your hair apply the mixture and rub it into your scalp. Leave it on for 10 minutes, then shampoo your hair as usual.

•To rinse your hair use 1/4 cup of vinegar mixed with 1/4 cup of water.

•Do not pick or scratch your scalp; it only makes the dandruff worse.

•Try to use a nonoily shampoo and wash your hair frequently. Use natural products that do not have any chemicals. Every time before washing your hair massage the scalp gently with your fingers.

•Avoid using soaps, greasy ointments and creams.

•Thoroughly rub a thick gel of aloe vera leaves into the scalp; leave overnight; shampoo in the morning.

•Apple cider vinegar will help restore the proper acid/alkaline balance of the scalp and kill a bacteria that clogs the pores that release oil to the scalp. The clogged pores result in scales and crusts being formed. Apply apple cider vinegar diluted 50% with water to the scalp and let dry. There is no need to rinse. Another similar remedy suggests pouring two tablespoons into a cup, applying the straight vinegar to the scalp, and leaving it on from 15 minutes to three hours before shampooing. Lemon juice may also be used. It is the acid in these remedies that helps bring the scalp back into chemical balance.

•Rub some pure coconut oil in your hair daily. The dandruff should clear up in a few days.

•Mix 7-10 drops with the normal amount of shampoo you use. Massage into your hair and leave on for at least 2 minutes. Rinse thoroughly with water, avoiding contact with eyes. See our Product.

•Listerine For mild cases of dandruff, use the mouthwash Listerine. It has antiseptic properties. Do not use on cases where the skin is broken as the Listerine can be irritating. It used to be advertised on the back of the bottle that Listerine cures dandruff.

•Combine olive oil and ginger root and apply to your scalp before shampooing. If your dandruff is really bad, put the mixture on 10-15 minutes before shampooing.

•Rub rosemary oil or a mixture of olive oil and crushed rosemary leaves into your scalp and leave on for 15 minutes.

•Make a tea of either sage or burdock and use as a rinse after shampooing.

•Make a rinse by boiling four heaping teaspoons of dried thyme in two cups of water for ten minutes; strain and allow to cool. Massage this tea in your clean, damp hair; do not rinse out. The oil from the thyme has antiseptic properties.

• A high sugar intake may be another major cause. Sugar requires B vitamins in order to metabolize and can cause a deficiency. To compensate take a high potency B-complex to relieve the dandruff. Related to the sugar problem is the fact that diabetes may be the cause of your dandruff. If you have diabetes the high sugar levels result in dehydration of the tissues as the body flushes out fluids in an attempt to rid itself of the sugar. One of the end results is dry skin.

• Shampooing in hot water may strip out the natural oils and dry out your scalp. Using cool water will close the pores and will relieve the flaking problem.

• People on low or no fat diets may be deficient in unsaturated fats called essential fats, such as omega-3 and omega-6 fatty acids.

• Blow-drying your hair may dry out the scalp and cause dandruff.

Hold your hair dryer at least 10 inches from your scalp.

Dry hair

Dry hair is a problem that develops from excessive exposure to the elements. Weather can damage and weaken the hair.

Sun, ocean water, sand, and wind dry out the scalp. Dry hair is very fragile and breaks easily especially when wet. Wet hair can stretch nearly double its length. This can be very damaging. If you have dry hair, try to brush it as little as possible when wet.

An oil treatment is recommended. This will help give your hair the natural oils that have been striped out of it and give thickness and shine. In this section you'll find a home made oil treatment for dry hair and a home made totally natural conditioner and shampoo for dry hair as well. We'll also show you how to incorporate sulfur into your diet and we'll share with you how French and Italians keep their hair healthy and shiny.

We recommend

•Use a mild shampoo containing fatty acids, protein, balsams, and moisturizers.

•Use only the amount recommended and do not repeat as this will remove too much natural oil from the hair.

•Milk and egg yolks have been used for many years to condition hair and add protein.

•Use conditioners that contain Comfrey. This herb is loaded with protein.

Essential oils for split ends.

10 drops of sandalwood essential oil.
10 drops of rosemary essential oil.
Mix the ingredients and rub them in using your fingers.

Hot oil treatment for dry hair.

2 ounces aloe vera gel.

2 ounces of castor oil.

6 drops of rose geranium cedar essential oil.

8 drops of rosemary essential oil.

2 drops of ginger essential oil.

Mix ingredients, warm oil and apply to hair and scalp in sections, cover the head with a towel and leave it on for 1 hour.

Castor oil washes easily from the hair but Italians have used olive oil for centuries.

•Garlic, onions, and all vegetables from the cabbage family are rich in sulfur.

Rinse for dry hair.

2 tsp. of comfrey essential oil.

2 tsp. of marshmallow essential oil.

2 tsp. of parsley essential oil.

2 tsp. of sage essential oil.

4 cups of water.

2 cups of vinegar.

Mix all the ingredients and use it to rinse your hair after shampooing. Keep it away from your eyes and catch the rinse in a bowl to be used for a second and third time.

Herbal conditioner for dry hair.

1 pint of water.

1 tsp. of burdock root.

1 tsp. of calendula flowers.

1 tsp. of chamomile flowers.

1 tsp. of lavender flowers.

1 tsp. of rosemary leaves.

1 tbs. of vinegar.

Boil water and pour over herbs. Steep for 20 minutes, strain and add vinegar. Apply after shampooing. Do not rinse out.

Oily hair

If the hair contains too much oil, it becomes sticky and lifeless and the oil collects dust and dirt which makes the hair dirty. All of these things cause dandruff.

Some people have the wrong idea that if you have oily hair you need a shampoo that removes the oil from the hair. This is not the right way to treat oil excess. The solution would be to use a mild shampoo, baby shampoo is a good alternative. Most shampoos have strong chemicals that strip oil completely. This causes the oil glands in the scalp to produce even more oil.

We recommend

•Add one of these essential oils to a small amount of shampoo: cedarwood, cypress, lemon, lemongrass, sage and patchouli. These herbs reduce the oil production by the scalp.

•Avoid putting protein and balsams on your hair. This increases oiliness.

Herbal shampoo.

2 ounces   unscented shampoo.

12 drops of chamomile essential oil.

12 drops of lavender essential oil.

Mix ingredients and shake well before use.

Herbal rinse for oily hair.

1 pint boiling water.

1 tsp. burdock root.

1 tsp. calendula flowers.

1 tsp. chamomile flowers.

1 tsp. lavender flowers.

1 tsp. lemongrass leaves.

1 tsp. sage leaves.

1 tbs. vinegar.

Pour water over herbs and steep for 20 minutes, strain and add vinegar. Rinse your hair with the preparation and don't rinse out. Henna protein super preparation.

2 cups warm water.

1 egg.

1 tsp. olive oil.

2 tbs. honey.

24 drops lavender essential oil.

3 ounces henna.

Mix all the ingredients and add them to henna, removing any lumps. Wet hair and apply the preparation from root to ends cover with a plastic bag and towel to keep body heat in. This breaks down the henna and makes the color darker. Keep it covered for 1 or 2 hours. Make sure the henna does not dry out. Rinse with warm water several times, follow with shampoo and conditioner.

IMPORTANT: Use gloves and an old T-shirt to avoid staining the skin.

Dermatitis:

As we all know, the skin is the largest organ in the body and the most visible, so any condition affecting it is impossible to ignore. The skin is not only exposed to cut, burns, bruises and scrapes, it can also develop diseases just like any other part of the body.

Dermatitis or Eczema is an inflammatory skin condition that produces blisters, redness, scaling, flaking, thickening, weeping, crusting, color changes and itching that can be very annoying. Many times Dermatitis is allergic in nature mainly by coming in contact with different materials, chemicals or plants, such as, rubber, latex, perfumes, gold, silver, poison ivy, soap, cosmetics etc.

People with thin dry skin are prone to develop dermatitis and other skin conditions. Another cause of dermatitis is sensitivity or allergy to some foods. Studies have shown that people with low stomach acid are sensitive to some types of foods thus making them prone to develop some kind of skin disorder.

People suffering from dermatitis are sensitive to some of the items listed above and should be mindful of their condition and avoid contact with any irritant. Prolonged exposure to the materials may worsen the symptoms and cause the dermatitis to spread.

Another type of eczema called atopic dermatitis (AD) affects the face, elbows and knees. It's extremely itchy. Also nummular dermatitis attacks arms and legs and produces circular lesions caused by contact with nickel.

We recommend

Skin wash.

Mix the following ingredients:

1 tsp. comfrey root.

1 tsp. white oak bark.

1 tsp. slippery elm bark.

2 cups of water.

Boil for 35 minutes use it to wash the affected area.

- Vitamin B complex is needed for healthy skin.
- Taking Biotin pills is essential to prevent dermatitis.

TIP: Did you know that foods containing raw eggs prevent biotin from being absorbed?

- Put Vitamin E on the affected area. It calms the itching.

- Take Zinc orally and apply it directly to the dermatitis.

- Shark cartilage reduces inflammation.

- Use a lotion made out of blueberry leaves. This is proven to be fantastic in relieving the inflammation of dermatitis.

- Rue contains flavonoids needed for inflammation reduction.

- Drink chamomile. It helps with inflammation.

- Make a paste mixing goldenseal root powder, Vitamin E oil and honey. Apply directly on the skin. This speeds up healing.
Skin Infection fighting tea.

Make a tea mixing:

1 tsp. burdock root.

1 tsp. Oregon grape root.

1 tsp. echinacea root.

1 tsp. yellow dock root.

3 cups of water.

Boil for 20 minutes, drink ½ a cup a day.

• Do not eat the following: eggs, peanuts, wheat, dairy products, sugar, strawberries, flour.

• Use a cream made with tea tree oil. It helps kill microbes and is a natural antiseptic.

Dermatitis skin treatment.

½ pau d'arco bark tincture.

½ goldenseal root tincture.

8 drops tea tree essential oil.

8 drops chamomile essential oil.

½ cups of olive oil.

½   ounce of dried comfrey leaves.

½   ounce dried calendula flowers.

½   ounce of pure beeswax.

4 drops lavender essential oil.

Heat the olive oil with comfrey and calendula in it for about 2 hours without making the oil boil. Strain while warm, add beeswax and heat enough to melt it. Add essential oils and tinctures and stir well. Apply as needed over the skin.

• A very powerful herb used to treat psoriasis and dermatitis is sarsaparilla, as published in the 1940's by the New England Journal of Medicine sarsaparilla was "dramatically" successful in treating these types of conditions.

Skin Poultice.

A poultice is very helpful prepared as follows:

1 tablespoon of dried coneflower flowers.

1 tablespoon of hyssop flowers.

1 tablespoon of goldenrod flowers.

1 tablespoon of dried sunflower petals.

Mix ingredients and soak them with boiling water, let cool, place between gauze and apply on the skin, remoistening as needed.

Natural Antiseptic spray.

1/8 tsp. lemon essential oil.

1/8 tsp. tea tree essential oil.

½ ounce goldenseal tincture.

½ ounce oregon grape root tincture or barberry bark tincture.

1 ½ ounces aloe vera.

Mix all the ingredients and shake well every day for a week. Place liquid in a spray bottle, shake well before use.

• Studies done in France on the herbs milk thistle and gotu kola have shown that these compounds greatly improve psoriasis and dermatitis. These herbs are being used in French hospitals in the form of salve and as an injection and people in that country have used them for many years to cure leprosy.

• Licorice is a very powerful herb to reduce the inflammation, and stress related to many types of dermatitis.

• The compound gamma linoleic acid (GLA) found in primrose oil reduces inflammation of the skin better then cortisone, as shown in a study done in 100 people.

Dermatitis tea.

½ tsp. sarsaparilla root.

½ tsp. licorice root.

½ tsp. burdock root.

½ tsp. pau d'arco bark.

½ tsp. bupleurum root.

3 cups of water.

Simmer for 10 minutes and steep for another 10 minutes. Strain and drink 3 cups a day.

• Take 500 milligrams of red clover 3 times a day.

Diabetes:

Diabetes is a disease that develops due to a problem with the hormone insulin, produced by the pancreas. Insulin controls the glucose in the blood and how much glucose is absorbed by the cells; which in turn use glucose to produce energy. When insulin is not present, or the body is not using it properly, glucose can't enter the cells and stays in the bloodstream producing hyperglycemia, or excess of sugar (glucose) in the blood.

There are two types of Diabetes, Type I and type II. In type I, the pancreas produces no insulin whatsoever, therefore the patient depends on insulin injection to control the glucose. This type of diabetes affects people less than 30 years old and develops when antibodies kill cells of the pancreas in charge of creating insulin. Type II diabetes develops in people 30 years of age and older and is caused by the insufficient or ineffective production of insulin. This type of diabetes can be controlled with drugs and proper diet. The symptoms for either type diabetes are hunger and thirst more then normal, weight loss, excessive urination, fatigue, the white part of the eye turns yellowish, one bruises easily and cuts take longer to heal.

If not managed properly diabetes can have very damaging results, such as, retinopathy, blindness, cardiovascular disease, amputation of foot or leg and kidney disease. Since Diabetes is so dangerous, it should always be monitored by a physician, but here you will learn how to manage your diabetes type II without synthetic drugs, using only herbs, vitamins and good nutrition.

Women may develop gestational diabetes during pregnancy due to the changes in the body while expecting. Although this condition disappears after delivery it is a clear sign that the woman is at risk for developing Type II diabetes later in life and is likely to suffer gestational diabetes in future pregnancies.

We recommend

• Take Alpha Lipoic Acid. It helps to control sugar level in the blood.

• Take 400 mcg. a day of Chromium Picolinate. It makes insulin more efficient helping keep sugar level low.

• Take Garlic in capsules. It helps circulation and regulates sugar level.

• 500 mg of L-glutamine and Taurine a day will reduce sugar cravings and to help release insulin.

• Take Vanadium. It helps insulin release glucose to the cells.

• Place 45 drops of ginseng tincture, 90 drops of Oregon grape root tincture and 1 ½ cups of warm water. Drink 1 cup in the course of the day.

- If you do not have high blood pressure you can take ginseng tea to lower sugar levels.

- A tea made with kidney beans, white beans, navy beans, lima beans, and northern beans removes toxins from the pancreas.

- Huckleberry promotes the production of insulin.

- Take Dandelion root to protect the liver.

- Eat Jupiter berries. They lower blood sugar levels.

- Eat a well-balanced diet, rich in fibers (raw vegetables and fruits).

TIP: Did you know that carrots raise blood sugar levels more than ice cream?

- If you are planning to get pregnant, be sure to control your diabetes months before you start trying. Should you become pregnant before it's managed, the baby could have birth defects in the first few weeks of pregnancy.

• Take good care of your feet. If you have diabetes, the nerves of the foot are the first part to get damaged, losing the sensation of pain; this is the main reason for foot amputation in people with diabetes.

• Wear comfortable shoes, with white cotton socks, keep them dry.

• If your child has diabetes make sure that his or her teacher knows exactly what the symptoms are, and what to do in case of poglycemia (too little glucose in the blood) and hyperglycemia (too much glucose in the blood).

Diarrhea:

When stools are loose and without consistency it is called diarrhea, an effective way for the body to get rid of an undesirable substance. This may be followed with symptoms like vomiting, stomach pain, thirst, fever, nausea and/or dehydration. In children and people 65 and older this may be dangerous.

Diarrhea and vomiting cause the loss of fluids which need to be replaced. In some cases diarrhea is the secondary symptom of another problem, but in most instances it is caused by food poisoning; bacteria in food or water; food allergies; or a virus. Also, excess alcohol consumption, laxatives and caffeine are known to cause diarrhea. Some medicines can trigger diarrhea, such as antibiotics (tetracycline, clyndamycin, penicillin). If you find, blood or mucus in the stool that is a sign of infection or parasites.

Some well-known drugs will stop diarrhea but they interfere with the natural process of cleansing that the body desperately needs. With natural remedies we may help ourselves feel better without stopping the immune system from doing its job.

Your body uses diarrhea to flush bacteria or viruses you might have ingested by eating bad food. Therefore, it might be a bad idea to stop diarrhea too quickly.   However, diarrhea does not work sometimes and if goes on for several days, dehydration and loss of important nutrients may occur which can be dangerous, especially in children. That's why we recommend the use of herbs instead of over the counter drugs. Using herbs you can stop diarrhea and target the cause of it at the same time.

FACT: The use of the vaccine against rotavirus has been stopped by the National Centers for Disease Control and Prevention and FDA for causing bowel obstruction.

We recommend:

• Take homeopathic Arsenicum if you feel you have eaten spoiled food. This will help control the discharge without interfering with the elimination of toxins.

- If you feel weak and have a burning pain in mid-section take cuprum arsenicosum .

Take 4 charcoal tablets every hour this will absorb the toxins from the body.

- Drink blackberry tea for mild diarrhea.

- Take cayenne in capsules.

- Wild oregano oil is an antibacterial, anti-parasitic and anti-viral.

- Ginger tea can stop cramps and pain.

- Drink plenty of fluids, but stay away from caffeine and alcohol. Drinks like ginger ale or carrot juice are good for making the stools less watery.

TIP: Do not drink apple juice this will make diarrhea worse.

• Boil brown rice and water for 45 minutes eat the rice (it contains Vitamin B) and drink the water.

• Do not eat dairy products. When suffering from diarrhea the body loses the enzyme needed to digest lactose.

• The homeopathic remedy Sulfur is excellent for diarrhea.

• Take charcoal tablets every 4 hours to absorb toxins.

Blackberry remedy.

1 tbs. chamomile tincture.

1/4 cup of blackberry brandy.

3 drops of ginger essential oil.

2 drops of peppermint essential oil.

Mix ingredients and shake well. Take 1 tablespoon every hour.

Blueberry remedy.

4 tbs. of dried blueberries.

1 pint of water.

Mix and boil the ingredients, simmer for 20 minutes, strain and drink

4 tablespoons every hour.

Traveler's remedy.

1 ounce quassia bark tincture.

1 ounce goldenseal root tincture.

½ ounce yerba santa leaves tincture.

½ ounce peppermint leaves tincture.

Mix this very bitter remedy and take 1 teaspoon 30 minutes before

meals as a preventive treatment. If already ill, double the dose.

Rice preparation for diarrhea.

½ cup of rice.

2 cups of water.

1/4 tsp. oregon grape root powdered.

½ tsp. cinnamon powder.

1 banana.

Boil rice and water until soft, (30 minutes). Blend rice oregon root powder and banana. Serve and sprinkle cinnamon on top. Rice and banana help stop diarrhea and return important nutrients lost.

Eye problems:

In this section:

Conjunctivitis

Bloodshot Eyes

Cataracts

Glaucoma

Retinopathy

The eyes are two of the most complicated organs in the human body. They are a very important part of our day to day life and there are several conditions that can affect the eyes. We all have experienced at one time or another some type of eye problem such as irritation, dryness, red eye, or some more serious conditions like cataract or blindness.

Although most of the time eye problems are localized or within the eye itself, the eyes also reflect diseases elsewhere in the body; for example blured vision can be a sign of diabetes, yellow eyes can be a clue to hepatitis and a marked difference in the pupil's size can indicate that a tumor is developing somewhere in the body.

We take for granted the power of vision and the complexity of the whole process. The eye ball is a sphere measuring about one inch in diameter coated with a white substance called sclera commonly known as the "white of the eye". Under the sclera is a network of blood vessels called choroid.

The part of the eye that we see from outside is covered with the cornea and in the center is the iris which can have several different colors. It gives us our eye pigmentation or "eye color". In the center of the iris is the pupil which is in charge of letting light inside the eye. Behind the iris (going inside the eye) are the lens and the retina which are sensitive to the light let in by the pupil. The retina is connected to the optic nerve and this one is connected to the brain.

There are six muscles outside the eye in charge of moving the eye (left, right, up and down) and other muscles inside the eye are in charge of focusing the lens so you can see far away or closer. There are also fluids that fill the eyeball and lubricants called tears that clean and protect the front of the eye.

But how does everything work?   The action of seeing something is very complex and amazingly fast. First, light enters the eye through the pupil which contracts and expands depending on the amount of light in the environment.

We need light in order to see, therefore, the pupil expands in darkness to allow more light to go in the eye. When too much light is in the environment, the pupil contracts to let less light in. As it enters the eye, the lens focuses light by thickening or thinning its size. Once focused, the light is transferred to the retina which in turn builds an image by using pigments. After the image is formed, it's sent through the optic nerve to the brain where the image is interpreted and analyzed.

To all this we have to add the other eye and the work that is performed by both eyes together which gives us the ability to see and judge distances, speed and movement so obviously these organs are very complex and important and any interference, in any of the steps mentioned, can result in a vision problem.

Many eye conditions can be prevented with proper diet and herbs.

Conjunctivitis

Conjunctivitis or "pink eye" is an inflammation of the conjunctiva which is the membrane that covers the entire eyeball and the inside of the eyelids. The symptoms of conjunctivitis are redness, eye pain, burning, blured vision, feeling of dryness and discharge of a sticky fluid.

Conjunctivitis is very contagious. Wash your hands and do not touch the affected area.

We recommend

Mix 2 tsp. chamomile flowers.

1 tsp. Oregon grape root.

2 cups of boiling water.

Let it sit for 20 minutes, cool, strain and use an eyewash.

• Use calendula in bacterial or viral conjunctivitis to reduce itching and inflammation, heal and soothe. It's an antiseptic perfect for irritation due to pollutants and allergies. Use it as a local compress and eyewash. It is available in eye drops as well.

• Use a lotion made out of Vitamin A and apply it directly.

• If the eye is swollen, peel a potato, cut it in thin slices and place them on eyes affected by conjunctivitis.

• Use Fennel. This plant although used in the kitchen for salads is also a very good herb for vision problems. When snakes shed their skin they are temporarily blinded and eat fennel to restore their sight. It can be eaten raw or made as a tea and the tea can be used as an eyewash.

• Use Eyebright herb in drops. It's excellent for conjunctivitis. This plant can be used internally and is much more effective than commercial eye drops and safer.

• Goldenseal is an anti-inflammatory and natural antibiotic. It kills many different kinds of bacteria and decreases swelling by removing fluid from tissues.

• Make a tea with goldthread. It treats inflammation of the conjunctiva and infection of eyes. It's also a good pain reliever. The tea can be used as an eyewash.

Bloodshot eyes

A bloodshot eye is a condition that develops when the small blood vessels that we see on the surface of the eye become inflamed with too much blood caused by insufficient oxygen to the cornea.
If overwhelmed with fatigue, eyestrain, alcohol consumption, insufficient Vitamin B2 and B6 or high blood pressure, bloodshot eyes may appear. However if all of these conditions are managed, bloodshot eyes should disappear.

We recommend

• Vitamin A is very necessary for a healthy vision.

• Eat spinach and take Lutein or spinach extract because they contain carotenoid needed for retina and eye tissue.

• Take a Vitamin B complex. About 100 mg. of each B vitamin 3 times a day has been shown to releive the B vitamin deficiency that leads to bloodshot eyes.

• Use raspberry leaves to make a tea and when cool, soak a piece of cotton and apply it to the eye.
• Using Eyebright herb in drops is excellent for bloodshot eyes. This plant can be use internally and is much more effective than commercial eye drops and safer.

• Cayenne it's an anti inflammatory for the mucus membranes Use very small amounts well diluted or in an eye drop form.

• Take Ginkgo biloba. It increases the delivery of oxygen and nutrients to the eye.

Cataracts

Cataracts are a clouding of the eye lens that causes blured vision, inability to focus and is progressive and painless. The cataract becomes thicker with time until it blinds the eye and is the number one cause of blindness in the world.

The most common type of cataract is senile cataract which means that it affects people 65 and older. This type of cataract is caused by free radicals that damage the lens.

TIP: Frequent x-ray causes the formation of chemical reactive fragments in the eye and this leads to cataracts

We recommend

Mix 1 cup of rose petals.

4 tbsp. of raspberry leaves.

4 cups of boiling water.

Let the ingredients rest for 30 minutes, strain and use as eye wash.

• Using Eyebright herb in drops is excellent for cataracts. This plant can be used internally and is much more effective than commercial eye drops and safer.

• Eat spinach and take Lutein or spinach extract because they contain carotenoid needed for retina and eye tissue and sometimes reverses cataracts.

• Vitamin A is very necessary for a healthy vision.

• Dusty miller is used to dissolve cataracts and corneal opacities if used in the early stages of the disease.

• Take Ginkgo biloba because it increases the delivery of oxygen and nutrients to the eye and clears toxins.

• Eat lots of green vegetables, especially spinach and, kale as well as berries, blueberries, blackberries, cherries and fruits rich in Vitamin C and E.

• Avoid dairy products and saturated fats as these produce free radicals which cause cataracts and damage to the lens.

• Do not use any antihistamines if you have cataracts.

• Bilberry Strengthens and protects veins and blood vessels, protects the retina, reduces pressure in glaucoma and can stop the growth of cataracts.

Glaucoma

Glaucoma is a very serious disease that affects the optic nerve. The pressure inside the eye rises, damaging the nerve and causing vision loss and blindness. People more than 65 years of age are at risk and people with diabetes as well.

This condition produces no symptoms.   Therefore, people who suffer glaucoma do not find out until it's very advanced.

Glaucoma has probably many causes. Some scientists claim it is related to stress, poor nutrition and high blood pressure. Collagen deficiency has been linked to glaucoma.

We recommend

• Take 50 mg. of Rutin 3 times a day. This bioflavonoid reduces pain and pressure inside the eye.

• Vitamin A and carotenoid are needed to keep healthy eyes and to improve night vision.

• Eat spinach and take Lutein or spinach extract because they contains carotenoid needed for retina and eye tissue and sometimes reverses many eye conditions.

• Eyebright herb in drops is excellent for glaucoma. This plant can be use internally and is much more effective than commercial eye drops and safer.

• Take Ginkgo Biloba because it increases the delivery of oxygen and nutrients to the eye and it clears toxins. Mix it with zinc sulfate to slow down progressive vision loss.

• Cayenne is an anti-inflammatory for the mucus membranes. Use very small amounts, well diluted with water or in eye drop form. It increases blood flow to the eye.

• Take Vitamin E. It removes particles from the eye lens.

• Bilberry strengthens and protects veins and blood vessels, protects the retina, reduces pressure in glaucoma and can stop the growth of cataracts.

• Use Coleus dropped directly into the eye to increase blood flow to the eye and decrease intraocular pressure.

• Use Fennel. This plant although used in the kitchen for salads is also a very good herb for vision problems. When snakes shed their skin they are temporarily blinded and eat fennel to restore their sight. It can be eaten raw or made as a tea and the tea can be used as an eyewash.

• Jaborandi is a herb that grows in the rainforest. It's been used for about 120 years in patients with glaucoma because it contains pilocarpine.

• Although we do not recommend it, many studies have shown that marijuana can help reduce intraocular pressure but it is unknown how marijuana achieves this result.

Diabetic retinopathy

Diabetes can cause retinopathy, a condition that develops when tinny blood vessels connected to the retina begin to leak. Then more blood vessels grow in the affected area causing vision problems and blindness in thousands of people suffering diabetes.Since this disease causes no symptoms in the beginning it is very hard to diagnose until the condition is advanced.

We recommend

• Vitamin A and carotenoid are needed to keep healthy eyes and to improve night vision.

• Take Ginkgo Biloba to increase the delivery of oxygen and nutrients to the eye and to clear toxins. It is very helpful in retinopathy.

• Bilberry strengthens and protects veins and blood vessels, protects the retina, reduces pressure in glaucoma and damage cause by diabetic retinopathy.

• Grape seed extract contains procyanidins which strengthens retinal capillaries and prevents clots or bleeding, provides vital nutrients, increases night vision and slows eye ageing. It also prevents and treats retinopathy and arteriosclerosis in the eye.

• Eat spinach and take Lutein or spinach extract. They contain carotenoid needed for retina and eye tissue and sometimes reverses many eye conditions.

• We recommend that you check Diabetes for important herbs and nutrients needed for diabetes and to prevent diabetic retinopathy.

Fever:

Fever is an elevation in body temperature. It's the body's protective mechanism against infection. The elevation in temperature happens when our immune system is fighting off bacteria and viruses that could harm our body. Fever is our strongest weapon in the fight against infections or diseases.

Normal body temperature ranges from 97 to 99 degrees Fahrenheit but varies throughout the day. Usually it's lower in the early morning and higher in late afternoon. A fever is considered to be any temperature above 100 degrees Fahrenheit. One should be concerned when temperature rises above 102 degrees Fahrenheit for an adult and 103 degrees Fahrenheit for children.

Often, having a high temperature is helpful for the body; it's the way the body acts to destroy harmful microbes. In an adult temperature less than 103 degrees Fahrenheit encourage the body to create more immune cells. A fever of 104 or higher can be a risk for people with cardiac problems since it accelerates the heart beat making it work harder and can cause irregular rhythms, chest pain or even heart attack. When a person has had a fever of more than 106 degrees for a long period of time it can cause dehydration and brain damage.

Although vigorous exercise in which the muscles generate heat faster than the body can dissipate it can cause a temporary rise in temperature it is not considered fever.

We recommend:

• Drink as much water as you can in order to replace fluid loss. It will also help bring down body temperature.

• Rest as much as possible.

• Avoid sudden changes in atmospheric temperatures.

• Avoid eating solid foods until the fever is gone. You can replace the foods by drinking plenty of distilled water and/or juices.

• When you have fever do not take any supplement containing either iron or zinc. Taking iron causes great tension in a body that is fighting infection and zinc is not absorbed by the body when you have fever.

• Take cool baths. Fill a bath tub, submerge and lie down for approximately 5 minutes. Repeat as needed until the fever is down.

• If the fever does not exceed 102 degrees let it run its course. It helps the body fight infection and eliminate toxins.

• When a child has fever do not give them aspirin. Instead try to reduce the fever with cold baths.

• If a baby of 3 months or younger has 103 degrees or more, call your doctor. If a child with fever has also a stiff neck, swelling of the throat or disorientation, see a physician immediately as these symptoms may indicate meningitis.

• To reduce fever some beneficial herbs include Blackthorn, Echinacea, Fenugreek seed, Feverfew, Ginger and Poke root. Caution: Avoid Feverfew during pregnancy.

• Taking a tea or a hot steam bath made with Elderberry may help.

• If you develop an unusually high fever, sponge your face and forehead with lukewarm water. It will reduce the fever and you will feel more comfortable.

To reduce fever you can make this tea:

1 tsp. Echinacea root.

1 tsp. White willow root.

1 cup water.

Combine ingredients in a pan, cover and bring to a boil. Reduce heat and simmer for 30 minutes, cool and strain. Take half a cup up to 4 times a day.

Flu :

Influenza, most commonly known as "the flu" or "grippe", is caused by a virus that infects the upper respiratory tract. There are two types of influenza, type A and B. They infect the throat, nose, lungs bronchial tubes, and middle ear. There are vaccines for the flu but since there are so many viruses that can cause influenza (about 200) they are constantly mutating, making it very difficult to achieve success against these types of viruses.

The symptoms for influenza are similar to those of a common cold, body aches, cough, hot and cold sweat, fatigue, headaches, fever, nausea, vomiting, throat pain and lack of appetite. Colds last for a week but the flu can last for up to 12 days and after all symptoms have disappeared a persistent cough remains for another week. Influenza is one of the thousands of diseases that modern medicine has yet to find a cure for but herbs and natural remedies can relieve the symptoms.

TIP: Did you know that the Flu shot or vaccine is made from chicken embryos? If you are allergic to eggs avoid Flu shots.

The allergic reaction is worse than the flu symptoms. Besides,

the effectiveness of the vaccine is not very good either.

Do not buy any over the counter drugs to deal with this virus. Most of

the medications on the market today only suppress the symptoms

and block the self defense mechanism of the body making it more

difficult to recover.

TIP: Do not use Aspirin. This can irritate the mucus membranes.

We recommend

• Take Vitamin C to boost immune system and increase the number

of white blood cells.

• Take Zinc lozenges to boost the immune system as soon the

symptoms develop.

• Colloidal silver kills viruses.

241

• Take Garlic capsules to decrease the growth of the virus.

Make a tea mixing:

1 tsp. bayberry bark.

1 tsp. grated ginger root.

½ tsp. cayenne powder.

1 cup of boiling water.

Let it sit for 20 minutes.

• Take "cold and flu" tablets. This homeopathic preparation has helped people avoid getting infected with the flu virus by taking one tablet a day throughout the flu season.

• Arsenicum album is a great homeopathic remedy. Take it if you are thirsty but feel better drinking warm fluids, lack of appetite, body aches, and feel worse during the night.

• Take bryonia if you cough or have throat and chest pain, dry mouth and lips or are very thirsty.

• Take eupatorium perfoliatum if you have pain in your bones and eyeballs.

• Take Gelsemium if you have chills, aches, fever but are not thirsty.

• Nux vomica is used when a simple cold has developed into influenza.

• If the fever is too high, take catnip tea and ½ tsp. of lobeliatincture every 4 hours. Do not use if pregnant or breast-feeding and do not give to a child less than one year old.

• Cat's claw shortens the duration of the flu.

• Cayenne in powder form added to juice or soup is very helpful for cleaning of mucus from the system and for relieving congestion.

- For cough, place echinacea extract (alcohol free) and goldenseal in your mouth and hold it for a few minutes, then swallow. This will keep the virus from multiplying.

- Elderberry it's an antiviral.

- Take a very warm bath with eucalyptus oil in the water. This will relieve your congestion.

- Olive leaf extract kills all types of viruses including the flu virus.

- Drink lots of juices and eat chicken soup to avoid dehydration.

- Take echinacea. This herb is antiviral and antibacterial and speeds healing and boosts the immune system.

- Horseradish is another herb that many use in the kitchen but it also has excellent properties to treat sore throat and upper respiratory tract infections. It reduces fever and expels concentrations of mucus.

• Use kava kava as a gargle for soothing and analgesic pain relief. Helps insomnia caused by coughing and sore throat.

• Myrrh is an antiseptic and anti-inflammatory, very powerful and excellent for chronic sore throats. It acts also as an expectorant and decongestant. It helps cure gum disease.

• In Europe it is common to see singers use oregano oil to fight respiratory allergies, laryngitis and sore throat. They take it for it's antifungal and antibacterial properties.

• Sage is used to cure sore throat, stuffed nose, gingivitis and coughs. It   is a powerful antiviral, antibacterial and antifungal. Use as a gargle.

• Wild indigo is an antiviral and antibiotic for infections. It stimulates the immune system and cures chronic sore throats.

245

• Mullein coats the throat with a mucus-like film which helps reduce the burning feeling. It clears mucus and phlegm.

• Osha is an antiviral that works great in the first stages of the infection of colds and flu, sore throat and phlegm. It acts as an expectorant.

• Poke root relieves inflammation and infection. It reduces coughing, pain and burning.

Make a gargle tonic with:

1 cup of boiling water.

2 tsp. sage leaves.

salt.

Mix all ingredients and let them steep for 30 minutes, drain and use as gargle when needed.

Make your own cough syrup mixing:

1 tbsp. licoriceroot.

1 tbsp. of marshmallow root.

1 tbsp. of plantain leaves.

1 tsp. of thyme leaf.

4 tbsp. of honey.

4 ounces of glycerin.

2 drops of anise oil.

Place all herbs in a container with boiling water, let it simmer for 20 minutes, strain, add honey, glycerin and, if desired, anise. Take 1 tbsp. as needed. It will keep in the refrigerator for several months.

Caution: Do not give honey to a child less than 2 years of age. It can be very harmful to them.

Gallbladder Disorders

The gallbladder is a 3 to 4 inch-long pear-shaped organ located on the right side of the body, directly under the liver. One of the functions of the liver is to remove poisonous substance from blood so that they can be excreted from the body. The liver excretes all these gathered toxins in a digestive agent called bile. Bile also contains cholesterol, bile salts, lecithin, and other substances. The bile (about one pint of it every day) goes first to the gallbladder, which holds it until food arrives in the small intestine. The gallbladder then releases the bile, which passes through cystic and bile ducts into the small intestine. Ultimately, the toxins are passed out of the body through the feces.

Abnormal concentration of bile acids, cholesterol and phospholipids in the bile can cause the formation of gallstones. The presence of gallstones is known to doctors as cholelithiasis. It has been estimated that 20 million Americans have gallstones. In fact, one in ten people have gallstones without knowing it. However, if a stone is pushed out of the gallbladder and lodges in the bile duct, this can cause nausea, vomiting, and pain in the upper right abdominal region. These symptoms often arise after the individual has eaten fried or fatty foods.

Gallstones can range from the size of a tiny grain of sand to larger than a pea-sized mass. Seventy five percent of gallstones are cholesterol stones, with the remaining 25 percent being pigment stones. Pigment stones are composed of calcium salts. Although the cause of pigment stones is unknown, factors such as intestinal surgery, cirrhosis of the liver, and blood disorders can increase the rate risk.

The presence of gallstones creates a possibility that cystitis, inflammation of the gallbladder, may develop. This can cause severe pain in the upper right abdomen and/or across the chest, possibly accompanied of fever, nausea, and vomiting. Other symptoms of gallbladder disease include constant pain below the breastbone that shoots into the right or left shoulder and radiates into the back. The pain can last from 30 minutes to several   hours. The urine may be tea- or coffee-colored, and there may be shaking, chills, and a yellowish discoloration of the skin and eyes. Gallbladder attacks occur often in the evening and can take place sporadically. Abdominal pain that occurs on a daily basis may be a problem unrelated to the gallbladder. A gallbladder attack may mimic a heart attack, with severe pain in the chest area.

Inflammation of the gallbladder requires immediate treatment. If left untreated, it can be life threatening.

We recommend

- Alfalfa cleanses the liver and supplies necessary vitamins and minerals. Twice a day for two days, take 1,000 milligrams in tablet or capsule form with a glass of warm water.

- Peppermint capsules are used in Europe to cleanse the gallbladder.

- If you have gallstones, or are prone to developing them, turmeric can reduce your risk of further problems.

- Other beneficial herbs include barberry root bark, catnip, cramp bark, dandelion, fennel, ginger root, horsetail, parsley and wild yam. DO NOT USE BARBERRY DURING PREGNANCY.

- If you have an attack, drink 1 tablespoon of apple cider in a glass of apple juice. This should relieve the pain quickly. If the pain does not subside, go to the emergency room to rule out other disorders such as gastroesophogeal reflux disease or heart problems.

Hair loss:

You could lose at least 100 of your 100,000 scalp hairs each day so you shouldn't be alarmed if this is the case with you. Usually, the lost hair is replaced by a new hair from the same hair follicle, located just below the scalp's surface. Luckily we have some great home remedies for hair loss in women to speed up growth.

Women also lose more hair as they age. Many experience a generalized thinning of the hair or a "widened part" in the center of the scalp after menopause. This is called female pattern baldness.

As with male pattern baldness, hormonal changes and genetic predisposition are to blame. Although they do not usually lose as much hair as men do, women are also constantly searching for a cure for this distressing problem. All in all, more than two-thirds of all men and women have some type of hair loss or thinning during their lifetime.

Premature hair loss or thinning can also be due to a wide variety of other causes. Most women lose quite a bit of hair in the two to three months after they deliver a baby, and this can continue for up to six months. One and a half to three months after severe stress, operation, infection, or high fever, a person may also lose a lot of hair. Likewise, two to three months after crash dieting with insufficient protein intake, hair may come out in handfuls.

Many prescription drugs can cause reversible hair loss. Cancer patients treated with certain chemotherapeutic drugs may lose up to 90 percent of their scalp hair, but it eventually returns after their treatment is finished. Birth control pills that contain high levels of progestin also can cause hair loss.

Other possible causes of hair loss include trauma; syphilis; tumors; thyroid disease; connective tissue diseases; bacterial, fungal, or herpes infections of the scalp; improper hair care with tight hairstyles, over brushing, or overuse of dyes and permanents; and, in women, too-high levels of male hormones.

Many different nutrient deficiencies result in hair loss, including deficiencies of vitamins A, B6, B12, folic acid, biotin, vitamin C, copper, iron, and zinc. Hair loss can be a sign of vitamin A toxicity as well as deficiency. Vitamins B6, B12, folic acid, copper, and iron are necessary for the normal formation of red blood cells that supply oxygen to the hair shaft.

Copper also functions in the formation of hair pigmentation, so copper deficiency can also cause color changes in the hair. With vitamin-C deficiency, the hair splits and breaks easily, resulting in dry, kinky, tangled hair. Silica also is important for hair growth and strength. Vitamin E is also necessary for good scalp and hair follicle health.

There is also an immune problem known as alopecia areata, in which the hair suddenly comes out in totally smooth, round patches. This condition can cause a lot of pyschological stress. A person with alopecia areata can also lose hair from his or her eyelashes, eyebrows, beard, and the other hairy areas of the body.

Because a full head of hair is associated with virility, youth, and attractiveness, hair loss and thinning can have a huge negative psychological impact on a person. If you start losing more hair than normal, a dermatologist will try to identify the cause by taking a complete history doing blood tests, and examining your hair visually, under the microscope, with hair analysis, and, perhaps, with a scalp biopsy.

Home remedies for Hair loss in Women

Home remedies for hair loss in women #1:

A high-potency multivitamin and multimineral daily.

• Beta-carotene. Take 25,000 international units daily.

• Vitamin-B complex. Take a supplement containing 100 milligrams of most of the major B vitamins. Also take an additional 50 milligrams of biotin daily.

• Vitamin C. Take 1,000 milligrams twice a day.

• Vitamin E. Take 400 international units daily, with 100 micrograms of selenium to aid its absorption.

• Iron. Take 50 milligrams daily.

• Zinc. Take 50 milligrams daily, with food and with 2 milligrams of copper.

• Silica. Take 250 milligrams twice a day.

• Free-form amino acid complex. Take 2 grams (2,000 milligrams) three times a day, before or after meals.

Home remedies for hair loss in women #2: In addition to correcting any vitamin deficiencies, women whose hair loss is due to physical trauma, crash diets, or heavy menstrual periods can benefit from supplementation with a high-potency multivitamin and 50 milligrams of iron, together with 1,000 milligrams of vitamin C to boost iron absorption.

Home remedies for hair loss in women #3: Thinning hair can be a sign of poor nutrient absorption, which in turn can be due to an insufficient supply of stomach acid or bacterial overgrowth in the stomach. Taking one tablet of hydrochloric acid (HC1) and one digestive enzyme capsule after starting each meal, plus 1/2 teaspoon of powdered acidophilus dissolved in 2 ounces of water twice a day between meals, can aid in nutrient absorption.

• Inositol with choline has been found to stimulate hair regrowth in some people with nonscarring alopecia. Take 200 milligrams twice a day.

Home remedies for hair loss in women #4:

Saw palmetto is the first choice of many herbalists for male pattern bald ness. Saw palmetto blocks the formation of dihydrotestosterone, a hormone thought to kill off hair follicles and lead to androgenic alopecia. Take 160 milligrams twice a day.

DS Some people have had success using aloe. It is suggested that you apply the gel to the scalp every night before bed, and also take 2 tablespoons of aloe juice orally each day.

255

Home remedies for hair loss in women #5: Arnica can be applied to the scalp twice a day in the form of a cream, ointment, or hair rinse made from arnica tincture diluted with warm water. Arnica increases local blood circulation, and may thereby help promote hair growth.

Home remedies for hair loss in women #6: Arnica can be applied to the scalp twice a day in the form of a cream, ointment, or hair rinse made from arnica tincture diluted with warm water. Arnica increases local blood circulation, and may thereby help promote hair growth.

Home remedies for hair loss in women #7: Jojoba oil may help with hair loss when applied to the scalp.

Home remedies for hair loss in women #8: Emu oil, or kalaya oil, is recommended as a moisturizer and hair-root stimulant to promote hair growth.

Home remedies for hair loss in women #9: Licorice also contains a chemical that prevents testosterone from being changed to dihydrotestosterone. You can add licorice tincture or extract to your favorite shampoo.

Home remedies for hair loss in women #10: Rosemary has long been believed to keep hair healthy and lush. Add one part rosemary oil to two parts almond oil and massage the mixture into your scalp for twenty minutes a day.

Home remedies for hair loss in women #11: Sage has been believed for centuries to help prevent hair loss. Like licorice, sage extract can be added to your favorite shampoo. Or you can use double-strength sage tea daily as a hair rinse to encourage hair growth.

Home remedies for hair loss in women #12: Safflower is considered to be a good vasodilator. Massage your scalp with safflower oil for twenty minutes a day to increase local blood flow and stimulate hair growth In general, hair loss is a condition that reflects the level of health of the person. Although not a dangerous disease, millions of people are desperately seeking a cure for hair loss. Our society drives us to look healthy and young and hair loss damages our looks and our self-esteem, making us less sure of ourselves.

But why do some people suffer from hair loss and others enjoy a full head of hair throughout their lives? Usually we lose about 100 hairs per day after a few months, a new hair grows out of the same follicle. In some men the new hair is thinner than the one before and when this one falls the next one is even thinner until eventually the follicle stops producing hair.

Women also suffer from hair loss as they age and reach menopause although they don't lose as much hair as men. Childbirth can cause hair loss. Mothers usually lose a lot of hair during a 6-month period after giving birth. Other reasons for hair loss in men and women are; stress, infection, surgery, high fever, diets, over brushing, syphilis and tumors.

There are some drugs that claim to regrow hair but they only achieve mild results and are full of side effects, for example minoxidil (Rogaine) should not be taken by people with high blood pressure and it may cause acne on the forehead and back. Another is finasteride (Propecia) which can be taken orally (men only) and causes sex problems, rash and if handled by a pregnant woman, can cause birth defects in the genital area of the fetus.

We recommend

TIP: Did you know that the herb Sage used as a rinse restores color to gray hair better than advertised products?

• Take Vitamins A, B6, B12, Folic acid, biotin, and Vitamin C. **Caution:** Too much Vitamin A can cause hair loss keep your intake less than 100,000 IU daily.

• Take Silica in capsules once a day to make hair stronger and thicker.
• Rinse your hair with a mix of apple cider vinegar and sage tea to help hair grow.

• To improve blood circulation to the scalp take Ginkgo Biloba.

• Take Saw Palmetto herb to unblock hair follicles and heal the prostate (like the drug found in Rogaine) by decreasing residues of dihydrotestosterone (DHT) in the scalp. It is 3 times more effective then Proscar in healing the prostate. It may be 3 times better then Rogaine.

- Nettles can be used locally or internally to prevent baldness and stimulate hair growth because it contains high amounts of silica.

- Use Rosemary oil locally to stimulate hair growth. It improves oxygen delivery to the follicles.

- Neem has been used in ayurveda for hundreds of years to help hair growth. It thickens hair, heals follicles and cleans the scalp.

- Horsetail contains silica therefore promoting hair growth.

- A Chinese herb called Fo-Ti restores hair color and hinders production of DHT, stops hair loss and thinning hair and encourages hair growth.

- Tea tree oil kills bacteria and mites that attack the follicles and causes hair loss.

Mix 1 tsp. of cayenne.

1 tsp. of yucca root.

2 cups of boiling water.

Let it sit for 30 minutes then apply this topical solution on the scalp to promote blood circulation to the area and help prevent hair loss.

• Pygeum works in the same way Saw palmetto does by reducing DHT in the scalp and thus promoting hair growth.

• Avoid drugs such as Rogaine and Propecia. They have side effects and although they are allowed to advertise that they re grow hair, only a small percentage of people see acceptable results. Besides, they must be used for the rest of your life. As soon as you stop, the hair loss resumes and some people have reported loss of hair at a higher pace then before the treatment started.

• Use shampoos and conditioners containing silica and biotin extracts.

- Avoid hair sprays and gels.

- Do not brush your hair too much.

- When towel drying your hair, don't rub. Instead pat your hair dry gently.

Rosemary Hair Oil.

1/2 tsp. rosemary essential oil.

1/2 tsp. jojoba oil.

Mix ingredients in a blender and process until smooth. Apply on the scalp a leave it for a few hours before washing it off.

Hair Formula.

1 cup aloe vera gel.

4 tbs. apple cider vinegar.

1 tbs. nettle tincture.

1/2 tsp. vitamin E oil.

1/2 tsp. rosemary essential oil.

Mix ingredients in a blender and process until smooth. Apply a small amount on the scalp once a day.

Hemorrhoids:

Hemorrhoids are swollen anal varicose veins. These veins can become so stretched that they push with extreme force, then rupture and bleed. The hemorrhoids cause rectal bleeding, pain, burning, inflammation, irritation and itching since the swollen tissues are difficult to keep clean.

Hemorrhoids may be external or internal. The external hemorrhoids you can see and feel as a soft bluish-purple lump. The internal hemorrhoids you probably won't notice because they are usually painless. There is another type of hemorrhoid called prolapsed, it is an internal hemorrhoid that collapses and protrudes outside the anus accompanied by a mucus discharge and heavy bleeding. They can become thrombosed and are terribly painful. The most common cause of hemorrhoids is chronic constipation or congested liver.

Other factors that can cause or contribute to hemorrhoids include obesity, poor exercise, food allergies, lifting heavy objects and insufficient consumption of dietary fiber.

In pregnancy, women can develop hemorrhoids due to the pressure of the growing uterus on the mayor veins. Constipation in pregnancy can make hemorrhoids more painful. Straining during bowel movement puts a lot of pressure on the veins around the anus area. Hemorrhoids are also common after childbirth.

We recommend:

• Eat foods that are high in dietary fiber, like wheat bran, fruits and vegetables. Also eat apples, broccoli, carrots, Brazil nuts, green beans, guar gum, lima beans, oat bran, pears, beets, peas, whole grains, psyllium seed and foods in the cabbage family. It's the best treatment to prevent and treat hemorrhoids.

• To help bleeding hemorrhoids eat foods highs in Vitamin K, such as alfalfa, dark green leafy vegetables and black strap molasses.

• Drink plenty of fluids to help prevent constipation. Fluids are the best stool softener.

• Avoid fats, animal products, coffee, alcohol and hot spices. They are hard on the lower digestive tract.

• Take flaxseed oil daily. It helps soften stools. Take 1 or 2 tbsp. in the morning.

• Do not strain when moving the bowels. Do not sit on the toilet for more than 10 minutes at a time to prevent the blood from pooling in the hemorrhoidal veins.

• Take a hot bath for 15 minutes to help reduce swelling and ease pain. Do not add bath beads, oils or bubbles. They can irritate sensitive tissues.

• Avoid cleaning the anus with soap. It can cause irritation to the affected area.

• Do not sit on hard surfaces. That can make hemorrhoids more painful.

• When you lift any object, do not hold your breath. That puts enormous strain and pressure upon the hemorrhoidal vessels.

• Do not use rough toilet paper. Instead use baby wipes or a moistened toilet paper.

• Avoid sitting or standing for long periods of time.

• Apply Aloe Vera gel directly on the anus. It relieves pain and soothes the burning sensation.

• Use Bayberry, goldenseal root, myrrh, and white oak in a salve form to relieve pain in the hemorrhoids.

• Brew a strong, warm tea using Lady's mantle (yarrow) and apply it to the hemorrhoids with a cotton ball several times a day or as required.

• Apply Witch hazel with a sterile cotton pad 3 times daily to shrink the swollen veins.

• Take Buck thorn bark, collinsonia root, parsley, red grape vine leaves or stone root either in capsules or tea form. They are also good for the treatment of hemorrhoids.

• To keep the bowels clean use Cayenne (capsicum) or garlic enemas. They relieve pain caused by hemorrhoids.

• To help heal hemorrhoids use a peeled clove of garlic 3 times a week as a suppository. Or peel a raw potato and cut it into a small cone shaped piece and follow the same procedure.

• Take an infusion of Pilewort. If it doesn't help, in addition drink a tea made of Witch Hazel, Periwinkle or Tormentil. Also, you can apply Pilewort ointment on the affected area 2 or 3 times a day.

• Take Butcher's Broom. It reduces inflammation and helps increase circulation. Use also externally to reduce swelling.

• Use Comfrey as an ointment, powdered root or tea from the leaf or powder to soothe irritation. It also promotes healing of tissues and is an anti-inflammatory.

• Use Horse Chestnut. It shrinks hemorrhoids, reduces swelling, pain and itching. It also strengthens blood vessels, tones the veins and is an anti-inflammatory.

• Apply Mullein flower or infusion in the hemorrhoids to speed tissue healing. It is a soothing emollient for dry, sore and irritated hemorrhoids.

• Use Peony. It helps with burning, itching or irritated hemorrhoids or pain after stools. It also helps repair fissures, ulcers and fistula.

• Apply Plantain ointments directly on the hemorrhoid to relieve irritation and swelling. it shrinks swollen veins and decreases bleeding.

• Use Stone root. it relieves pain, itching and burning of chronic protruding or internal hemorrhoids. it also reduces bleeding and helps with chronic diarrhea or constipation.

• To reduce inflammation and encourage healing, make a small Witch Hazel compress and keep it on the affected area for as long as possible.

• Add Bayberry and Yellow dock (both astringent herbs) and add them to cocoa butter which can then be shaped into a suppository and placed in the anus.

• Make this tea or wash for hemorrhoids to relieve pain and help the affected area heal faster.

1 tsp. evening primrose

1 tsp. self- heal

1 tsp. peppermint leaves

1/4 water

Combine all the ingredients in a pan and boil until the liquid is reduced to 2 cups, then strain. Drink up to 2 cups a day.

Hemorrhoids Wash.

1 tsp. Blackberry leaves

1 tsp. Witch hazel leaves

1 tsp. mullein

2 cups boiling water

Combine all the ingredients in a nonmetallic container and cover with the boiling water, steep for 30 minutes, cool and strain. Use as wash whenever needed.

• Supplements are also important to prevent or cure hemorrhoids.

Supplements such as:

Calcium + Magnesium. It help prevent cancer of the colon and is essential for blood clotting.

Vitamin C + bioflavonoids with hesperidin and rutin speed healing.

Vitamin B complex + Vitamin B12 + choline and inositol reduce stress on the rectum and improve digestion.

Coenzyme Q10 helps heal faster and increases cellular oxygenation.

Potassium prevents constipation which can cause hemorrhoids.

Shark cartilage treats pain and inflammation.

Vitamin D3 aids in the healing of mucous membranes and tissues. It helps to absorb calcium.

• Here are some homeopathic remedies to cure hemorrhoids.

If the hemorrhoids are accompanied by aching in the lower back and at the base of the spine or a sensation in the rectum like splinters or sticks or a sensation of pressure in the rectum as if would protrude and there is little or no bleeding take Aesculus.

If you have a mild discomfort such as stinging pains, tight sensation or a constant uneasy feeling in the anal area which is worse in the morning, wearing tight clothes or is worse in cold or open air and there is a little or no bleeding or if you have itching in the anus and if you apply cold water you feel relief or you have chronic constipation, take Nux vomica. Also if the hemorrhoids appeared after overuse of laxatives, coffee, medications or drugs, take Nux vomica.

When itching is the predominant symptom or you have a burning or sore pain in the rectum and you feel better when applying cold water and you have diarrhea rather than constipation, take Aloe.

This remedy is ideal during the first 2 days of acute inflammation around the hemorrhoids. If you have too much redness and swelling and great pain and tenderness in the hemorrhoids, take Belladonna.

• If you can barely stand a very light touch on the inflamed hemorrhoid or if you see blood during a bowel movement and it feels better when applying warm water, take Muriatic acid.

• If you see a significant amount of dark, thick blood flow from the hemorrhoids and they are not tender to touch and you feel pulsation in the rectum, take Hamamelis.

• If you find relief applying cold pads and you feel thirst less and you don't want any clothes touching the hemorrhoids plus no two stools are alike in color or consistency, take Pulsatilla.

Caution: All the homeopathic remedies listed can be used by pregnant women, except Hamamelis.

Insomnia:

Insomnia is the inability to fall asleep or waking in the middle of the night and staying awake. If this problem continues for more than a month it is called chronic insomnia. Most of the cases of insomnia are related to normal day to day worries and tension or simply to caffeine consumption and is not a serious condition but it can be very frustrating and can cause lack of attention and bad temper.

Chronic insomnia is a different matter and it can interfere and disrupt a normal life. It contributes to headaches, dizziness, mental exhaustion, confusion, memory problems and emotional instability. Insomnia is not a disease but it can be a sign of a more serious disorder such as arthritis, asthma, stress, kidney, heart disease, etc.

TIP: Did you know that waking up at 1:00 to 3:00 a.m. is a sign of a liver dysfunction?

Many people turn to sleeping pills for help but this is hardly the answer to insomnia problems. These drugs cause a number of side effects including liver damage, high blood pressure and they weaken the immune system. Besides, one can very easily become dependent of them. Once they do, a higher dose is needed and when they are discontinued the use withdrawal symptoms become a major problem and insomnia resumes along with agitation and fogginess which causes people to reach for the pills again and in an even higher dose.

We are sure you will see that there is no need to put your body through pain caused by the side effects of these drugs, especially when there is a better answer in the form of natural herbs. Take a look.

We recommend

• Hops calms nerves, relieves tension and helps in cases of insomnia caused by stress, headaches and indigestion. It does not affect the early waking hours of the morning.

• A few hours before bedtime take Kava kava. It reduces stress, tension, anxiety and relaxes muscles. It helps you to fall asleep deeper and to rest more.   It can be used as a sedative when taking a large dose as effectively as benzodiazepines but without the side effects.

• The most popular herb for insomnia is Valerian. It relaxes nerves and muscles, improves sleep quality and makes falling asleep easier. Great for insomnia caused by mind activity, fear, fatigue or excitement. It's as good as many barbiturates but has no side effects or addiction.

Mix the following ingredients:

1 tsp. chamomile flowers.

1 tsp. hops.

1 tsp. valerian root.

1 cup of boiling water.

Steep for 45 minutes, strain and drink 1 hour before bedtime.

Make a tea mixing the following ingredients:

1 tbsp. of catnip leaves.

½ tbsp. of hops.

1 tbsp. of chamomile flower.

1 tbsp. of passionflower.

2 cups of boiling water.

Steep for 45 minutes, strain and drink 1 cup before bedtime.

• Catnip has sedative and tranquilizing properties. It is very good for insomnia caused by indigestion, gas, infant colic or menstrual cramps. It relaxes the body and mind during colds and flu.

• Passionflower helps if insomnia occurs from overwork, stress, pain, cough, drugs or alcohol. This is a great herb for children and infants teething, stomach pain etc. It soothes and relieves anxiety, irritability and is good for people with asthma or heart disease.

• Skullcap relieves insomnia caused by anxiety, worry or pain.

• Before going to bed, eat any of the following: bananas, milk, tuna, turkey, yogurt all of these contain tryptophan, it's been proven that they promote sleep.

• Avoid the following foods before bedtime: ham, cheese, chocolate, sausage, tomatoes, sugar.

• Do not use the bedroom for reading, watch TV, needle work etc. Go to the bedroom when you are sleepy or to for sex only.

• Jamaican dogwood is a strong pain reliever, sedative and antispasmodic. It's very helpful for muscular back pain, asthma, menstrual pain, insomnia, toothaches, and nervous conditions.

Sore throat:

A sore throat is a common and minor condition in which the back of the throat becomes irritated. Most cases (90% of them) are caused by a virus such as the one that causes colds and flu or the bacteria that cause strep infection. In cases of bacterial or viral infections antibiotics are completely ineffective and should not be taken.

Other causes of sore throat are: medication, surgery, radiation, dust, smoke, chemicals, loud talking, tooth and gum infection, allergies.

TIP: Did you know that mercury tooth filling can cause inflammation and ulceration in the mouth and throat?

In children a sore throat may be an indication of chickenpox or measles. Keep in mind other symptoms related to these diseases but remember that children show signs of a sore throat in many other illnesses.

We recommend

• Take echinacea. This herb's antiviral and antibacterial properties speeds healing boosts the immune system.

• Horseradish is another herb that many use in the kitchen but also has excellent properties to treat sore throat and upper respiratory tract infections. It also reduces fever and expels concentrations of mucus.

• Use kava kava as a gargle for soothing and analgesic pain relief. It also helps insomnia caused by coughing and sore throat.

• Myrrh is an antiseptic and anti-inflammatory that is very powerful and excellent for a chronic sore throat. It also acts as an expectorant and decongestant and helps cure gum disease.

TIP: Store your toothbrush in grapefruit seed extract to kill germs and bacteria. If you used hydrogen peroxide, wash the brush before using.

• In Europe it is common to see singers use oregano oil for its antifungal and antibacterial properties to fight respiratory allergies, laryngitis and sore throat.

• Sage is used to cure sore throat, stuffed nose, gingivitis and coughs and is a powerful antiviral, antibacterial and antifungal. Use as a gargle.

• Wild indigo is an antiviral and antibiotic for infections. It stimulates the immune system and cures a chronic sore throat.

• Mullein coats the throat with a mucus like film helping reduce a burning feeling. It clears mucus and phlegm.

• Osha is an antiviral that works great in the first stages of an infection such as colds, flu, sore throat and phlegm. It acts as an expectorant.

• Poke root relieves inflammation and infection and reduces coughing, pain and burning.

Make a gargle tonic with:

1 cup of boiling water.

2 tsp. sage leaves.

salt.

mix all ingredients and let it steep for 30 minutes, drain and use as gargle when needed.

Make your own cough syrup mixing:

1 tbsp. licorice root.

1 tbsp. of marshmallow root.

1 tbsp. of plantain leaves.

1 tsp. of thyme leaf.

4 tbsp. of honey.

4 ounces of glycerin.

2 drops of anise oil.

Place all herbs in a container with boiling water, let them simmer for 20 minutes, strain, add honey and glycerin and, if desired, anise. Take 1 tbsp. as needed. Keeps in the refrigerator for several months.

TIP: Did you know that sore throat can be contracted from bacteria in toothbrushes?

Caution: Do not give honey to a child less then 2 years of age. I it can be very harmful to them.

Make your own sore throat tea by mixing:

1 tsp. Canadian fleabane leaves.

1 tsp. slippery elm bark.

1 tsp. echinacea root.

2 cups of boiling water.

Step for 30 minutes, strain, drink it warm up to 2 cups a day.

Make your own sore throat gargle by mixing:

1 tbsp. of elderberry fruit juice.

1 tbsp. of sumac extract.

1 tsp. echinacea root extract.

Use as gargle as needed.

Heartburn:

Heartburn is a burning sensation and pain in the stomach and chest behind the breastbone. The symptoms of heartburn are the following: bloating, gas, nausea, shortness of breath and/or an acidic or sour taste in the throat and mouth.

Heartburn is caused when hydrochloric acid which is used to digest food is released up the esophagus. On its way up the acid irritates the sensitive tissues in the esophagus and throat. Usually the esophageal sphincter muscle contracts thus preventing the stomach acid from shooting up into the esophagus but if this muscle is not functioning properly the acid can slip past it and this is when heartburn symptoms start. It is called Gastroesophageal reflux disease because of the muscle malfunction but it's also known as dyspepsia, chronic heartburn or acid indigestion. If left untreated the repeated flow of acid through the esophagus can scar and produce changes in the cells lining and can cause cancer later in life.

A hiatus hernia develops when the stomach bulges up into the diaphragm. This condition can also cause heartburn. Other triggers for heartburn are alcohol drinking, smoking and eating acidic foods.

The good news is that herbs can deal with this problem very easily.

TIP: Doctors no longer recommend drinking milk to reduce

heartburn. It has been proven that milk temporarily reduces the symptoms only to increase acid production by the stomach which causes more heartburn.

If you are one of those people who uses antacids, think about this next time you are about to take one. Antacids reduce nutrient absorption such as Iron and increase blood pressure. They also upset the kidneys and their relief is short.

The best solution for heartburn is the use of herbs and vegetables.

We recommend:

• Papaya chewable tablets can be purchased in health stores and they are helpful reducing heartburn.

• Drink Aloe Vera juice to heal the intestinal tract.

• Drink Chamomile tea after meals to relieve esophageal irritation.

• Doctors are using Licorice to treat heartburn and stomach and esophagus ulcers.

• Drink a large glass of water at the first sign of heartburn. If the symptoms are not too strong this will help.

• Make a juice using raw potatoes. Wash the potato very well do not peel it, just place it in the juicer, mix it with some other juice for taste and drink immediately after juicing.

• For people suffering from severe cases of heartburn or gastroesophageal disease, it is recommended that they eat lots of raw vegetables, smaller portions and chew slowly and completely before swallowing.

• Papaya seeds and pineapple aids digestion.

• Do not eat and go to bed because this increases the chance of developing heartburn. It is recommended to wait three hours after a meal before going to sleep.

• Avoid caffeine, fried foods, fats, tobacco, tomatoes, onions, and spicy foods if you suffer from heartburn.

• Remember that heartburn can be triggered by anger and stress.

• Anise improves appetite and helps digestion if taken after meals. Very helpful in heartburn, reduces infant colic, nausea, gas and cramps.

• Geranium relieves pain and acidity and accelerates healing of bleeding ulcers.

• Meadowsweet reduces stomach acidity, heartburn and nausea and aids ulcers and controls gastritis and diarrhea.

• Ginger relieves indigestion and gas and prevents and heals ulcers and reduces heartburn.

Heartburn preparation.

1 tsp. Chamomile flowers.

1 tsp. Lemon balm leaves.

1 tsp. Licorice root.

½ tsp. Slippery elm bark.

½ tsp. Fennel seeds.

½ tsp. Catnip leaves.

1 ½ cups boiling water.

1 ½ cups apple juice.

Mix herbs and cover with water. Steep for 20 minutes, strain and add juice. Drink 2 cups a day.

Gastritis

Gastritis means "inflammation of the stomach." In most cases the lining of the stomach suffers erosion and perforations, sometimes even bleeding. The most common causes of gastritis are alcohol and most pain killers. From aspirin, Advil, Motrin and Nuprin to Aleve and many others cause irritation of the gastrointestinal tract and this leads to gastritis and ulcers.

People suffering from stress are also prone to gastritis. Surgery, burns, trauma and other serious medical problems increase the chances of developing gastritis.

The way gastritis attacks the stomach walls is by disrupting the mucosa, the name given to the lining of the stomach. However, other types of gastritis produce inflammation underneath the stomach lining due to bacteria or anemia.   These cases are prone to develop into ulcers.

Gastritis in most cases is painless. Common symptoms are: loss of appetite, vomiting, nausea, bloating and indigestion and some people may experience abdominal pain when eating.

We recommend:

• Eliminate dairy products from your diet until the digestive system is healed.

• Drink eight large glasses of water a day.

• Take 400 IU a day of vitamin E to reduce inflammation in the stomach.

• If your gastritis is caused by anemia, take supplemental

chlorophyll two capsules three times a day and follow the recommendations under anemia.

- Licorice (DGL) helps heal the gastrointestinal tract. Chew 300 to 600 mg. 30 minutes before meals. This herb is also used to treat ulcers. Licorice is as effective as Tagamet.
- Take Artichoke if you feel abdominal pain, bloating or to relieve vomiting and nausea.

TIP: Do not use cayenne in acute cases of gastritis or ulcers.

One of the best herbs for treating gastritis is Ginger. It relieves almost all symptoms including indigestion and gas, quickly healing stomach and intestinal tissue and reduces inflammation and ulcerated linings. Ginger is an anti-inflammatory and antibacterial. It reduces nausea, stimulates digestion of fats and it's a natural antibiotic.

• Goldenseal destroys bacteria that causes gastritis, stomach inflammation and ulcers.

• Marshmallow relives nausea, indigestion, gastritis and ulcers.

• Peppermint contains volatile oils like menthol. It relieves indigestion, gastritis and stomach ulcers.

• Papaya seeds and pineapple aid digestion. It should be eaten slightly ripe. Papaya is rich in digestive enzymes.

Peptic Ulcer

A peptic ulcer is an area of erosion in the mucous membranes of the stomach or duodenum, the upper portion of the intestine directly below the stomach. Ulcers are in part caused (and can be worsened) by the corrosive action of the gastric acids. Gastric juices are part hydrochloric acid and part pepsin, an enzyme that helps break down food. The walls of the stomach secrete a mucus substance to protect the linings from the corrosive action of the stomach acid. However if there is too much acid or not enough mucus coating the walls of the stomach, a peptic ulcer may develop. External substances can also irritate the linings of the stomach, things like tobacco, alcohol and some drugs like Advil, Aleve, Aspirin, Motrin, etc. are also part of the ulcer causing irritants.

It's now known that a bacterium called H. pylori can also contribute to the development of ulcers. This type of bacterium is commonly found in the linings of the stomach and is the principal cause of ulcers. It has been shown that 90% of people suffering from ulcers in the duodenum and 75% of all gastric ulcers are caused by this bacteria which attacks the walls of the stomach and has been linked to gastric cancer as well.

Ulcers are very common in the bottom part of the stomach and upper part of the duodenum and men are more likely to develop ulcers than women.

The symptoms of peptic ulcers are very different from person to person. Some feel a burning pain in the stomach and others feel it in the chest. Most people feel better during meals and other feel worse eating. In any case the pain may be severe enough to cause insomnia and can be triggered by stress.

We recommend:

• It's very important to follow a diet rich in fiber and low in fats. Eat steamed green vegetables like alfalfa, broccoli and tomatoes.

TIP:Did you know that deficiency in vitamin K has been linked to ulcers?

Vitamin K prevents bleeding and promotes healing.
Our body produces enough of this vitamin but people with

deficiency are prone to develop ulcers. Vitamin K is found in tomatoes, cheese, egg yolks, liver and in most green leafy vegetables.

• Eat small portions to avoid producing too much digestive acid but eat frequently to keep these acids from attacking the stomach linings.

• Studies have shown that cabbage juice cures ulcers in less that ten days. Prepare cabbage juice and drink one quarter a day divided in four doses (must be taken immediately after juicing). If you can't tolerate the taste or odor of cabbage there is a Chinese remedy made with dried cabbage that has been used for many years with excellent results.

• For bleeding ulcers eat organic baby food and drink brown rice water to soothe the digestive system.

• Avoid milk. Although it soothes the digestive tract and neutralizes stomach acid, it also stimulates the production of more acid further irritating the ulcerated area.

• Avoid coffee, alcohol, citrus juices, sugar and hot and spicy foods. These substances irritate the stomach and encourage the production of gastric acid.

• Take 5000 IU of vitamin A four times a day for six weeks to heal the mucus membrane.

• Take vitamin E to heal the stomach linings.

• Drink 1/4 cup of aloe vera juice a day. It's been used for centuries to relieve the symptoms of ulcers.

• Goldenseal is a natural antibiotic. Take 500 mg. of standardized extract.

• Licorice (DGL) helps heal the gastrointestinal tract. Chew 300 to 600 mg. 30 minutes before meals. This herb is also used to treat ulcers. Licorice is as effective as Tagamet.

• The homeopathic remedy carbo vegetabilis reduces the production of stomach acids and relieves the discomfort. Take 30x or 15c as needed.

• Papaya seeds and pineapple aid digestion. It should be eaten slightly ripe. Papaya is rich in digestive enzymes.

• Marshmallow relives nausea, indigestion, gastritis and ulcers.

• Stomach acid Self-Test.

If you suffer from stomach pain there is a way to find out if the problem is caused by excessive amounts of gastric acids. At the first sign of pain, swallow a tablespoon of apple cider vinegar or lemon juice. If this gets rid of the pain, you most likely have too little stomach acid but if the pain gets worse then you have too much acid and the recommendations above will help you correct the problem.

• Garlic kills bacteria and microbes and it aids the rapid healing of ulcers.

Ulcer Pain Night Reliever.

Mix the following herbs.

1 tsp. Licorice DGL extract.

1 tsp. Hops.

1 tsp. Passionflower.

1 tsp. Skullcap.

1 tsp. Valerian root.

2 cups boiling water.

Strain the herbs and let the liquid cool, Hot liquids can irritate the linings and make the symptoms worse. Drink one cup after dinner. It will reduce pain and improve sleep.

NOTE: Prescription and over the counter drugs do relieve temporarily the symptoms of ulcers but they don't treat the root of the problem. Ulcers are damaged tissue that needs to be repaired. Ulcer drugs create the illusion that the condition has been cured and this leads the person to believe that it's ok to go back to their old diets and habits. In the long term this can prove to be fatal. Many cases of stomach cancer are the result of poorly treated ulcers.

Stress:

Stress is the body's reaction to a physical, emotional, social

or mental condition imposed on the person. These changes, whether

good or bad, produces tension or stress. There is no way to avoid

stress completely. Injuries, weddings, meetings, childbirth, deadlines,

bills to pay, even going to a party is stressful.

It's part of our daily life and is very hard to control but there are

situations in life that create an extraordinary amount of stress, things

like overwork, death of family or friends, surgery etc. which in turn

can be damaging to our health leading to fatigue, headaches,

backaches, muscle pain, stiff neck, loss of appetite, memory loss, low

self-esteem, lower sexual drive, changes in sleep patterns and

shallow breathing. Adding all of these up results in a potential chance of becoming ill with an even more severe condition, things like high blood pressure, skin disorders, heart attacks, cancer and obesity.

We recommend

Mix 1 tsp. of valerian rhizome.

1 tsp. of licorice root.

1 tsp. of siberian ginseng root.

1 tsp. of kava root.

Take one teaspoon every 3 or 4 hours.

• Take Ashwaganda. This herb comes from India, improves mental and physical performance, relaxes brain waves and reduces stress, especially in people affected by overwork, anxiety, sexual debility and fatigue.

• Ginkgo biloba improves circulation and brain activity.

• Licorice protects against damaging effects of stress, increases energy and reduces inflammation to boost the immune system.

- Siberian ginseng stimulates the immune system and gives more stamina, alertness and resistance to stress induced illness.

- Holy basil lowers stress, blood pressure and blood sugar levels. It invigorates and increases vitality.

- Ginseng reduces fatigue and regulates sleep. It controls stress from mental and physical overload and improves concentration.
- Cordyceps promotes immunity, sex drive, improves endurance, vitality and reduces exhaustion.

- Schizandra counters the effects of stress and fatigue and improves your ability to do mental and physical work.

- Kava kava relaxes the brain and body.

- St John's Wort is a good antidepressant and calms nerves.

Mix 1 tsp. of kava kava root.

1 tsp. of hops.

1 tsp. dried skullcap.

1 cup of boiling water.

Let it sit for 1 hour. Strain and drink 1 tablespoon every 3 to 4 hours.

Mix 2 tsp. of valerian root.

1 tsp. of peppermint leaves.

1 cup. boiling water.

Steep for 45 minutes, drain and drink 1 cup per day.

• Using some or a combination of herbs we have mentioned will make you sleep better at night this is very important to achieve. Not enough sleep is one of the first symptoms that must be dealt with in order to fight stress.

• Jamaican dogwood is a strong pain reliever, sedative and antispasmodic. It's very helpful for muscular back pain, asthma, menstrual pain, insomnia, toothaches, and nervous conditions.

Things we can do to avoid stress and better our lives.

Learn to relax. Many times relaxing our body leads to relaxing of the mind.

Do not eat or drink too much caffeine. Although it gives you stamina and vitality, it also disturbs sleep patterns and makes you more nervous.

When things are not going the way you want, don't "talk down on you" the way you talk to yourself has a lot to do with the way you feel. Things like "I'll never learn this," "I can't do it"   or "I hate this guy" are negative thinking and promotes stress, depression and frustration.

Take warm baths using essential oils. (Aromatherapy).

Find a hobby, something you like to do and spend time for yourself.

Take a weekend off, but don't stay home, drive to another town or to a quiet place.

Tonsillitis

Tonsillitis is an inflammation of the palatine tonsils, which are the accumulations of lymphatic tissue on the right and left sides of the upper throat. It can be caused by either viral or bacterial infection. Generally, younger children tend to get viral tonsillitis, while older children and adults tend to get bacterial tonsillitis (caused by Streptococcus bacteria). Symptoms include sore throat, difficulty swallowing, hoarseness, coughing, redness, pain and swelling. If the cases of tonsillitis are severe other symptoms may appear, like, headaches, earaches, fever, chills, nausea, vomiting, and enlarged lymph nodes in different parts of the body.

In adults this condition may be a sign of a depressed immune system resulting in the inability to fight infections and other diseases. Also improper diet (too high in refined carbohydrates and low in protein and other nutrients) may predispose one to develop tonsillitis. In some cases this condition becomes chronic, due to the repeated bouts. If left untreated tonsillitis can lead to a more sever illness called Peritonsillar abscess in which the airways become obstructed making breathing difficult. After repeated bouts the infection can spread to the neck and chest making it hard to treat. Also, scar tissue grows every time the tonsils become inflamed aggravating the symptoms and the annoyance.

A person suffering from this disease should first boost his or her immune system and then attempt to treat the condition, always as naturally as possible.

We recommend

• Take vitamin C w/ bioflavonoids 5,000 - 20,000 mg daily to fight infection and boost immune system.

• Echinacea fights infection and boosts the immune system; take as much tea as you can or take 1/2   a teaspoon twice a day of tincture.

• Pau d'arco is a natural antibiotic that improves the immune system and is also a powerful antioxidant. (see antioxidants).

• Chamomile reduces headaches, fever and pain.

Tonsillitis Pain reducer Tea.

1 tsp. elder flowers.

1 tsp. peppermint leaves.

1 tsp. yarrow.

4 cups of water.

Boil water and remove from heat, place herbs in the water and steep for 20 minutes, strain and drink 2 cups a day.

- Flaxseed oil reduces pain and inflammation and speeds recovery.

- Place a poultice made with Hot Mullein to soothe.

- Marshmallow tea coats inflamed mucous membranes. Mix 3 tablespoons of marshmallow blossoms and 3 cups of cold water, steep for 12 hours then heat and strain. Drink 2 or 3 cups a day.

Tonsillitis Gargle remedy.

2 tsp. sage.

1 tsp. alum.

4 cups of water.

Boil water and herbs and steep for 45 minutes, strain and add 5 drops of peppermint. Mix well   and use it as a gargle as many times as needed.

• For a sore throat take goldenseal extract or St. John Wort extract. Six drops a day for no more than 5 days.

• Thyme reduces fever, headaches and mucus. It's very good for treating chronic respiratory problems and sore throat.

• Salt water gargles also help reduce inflammation and irritation of the throat.

• Remember that cigarette smoke irritates the mouth and throat.

Tonsillitis Steam Treatment.

Place   3 drops of lavender essential oil

3 drops lemon essential oil.

3 drops bergamot essential oil.

3 drops tea tree essential oil.

In 1 quart of boiling water. Place a towel over your head, lean close to the steam and inhale with your eyes closed. The fumes from the oils will relieve pain.

Wrinkles:

Wrinkles form when the skin thins and loses its elasticity. The appearance of some wrinkles is due to aging and is the most common skin problem for women. One of the first signs of wrinkles normally appear around the eye and is called " crow's feet." As time goes by the cheeks and lips are the next thing we notice. As we age, our skin becomes thinner and dryer, both factors contribute to the formation of wrinkles.

There are many factors that can contribute in the development of wrinkles some of which are: diet and nutrition, muscle tone, pollution, habitual facial expressions, chemicals, stress, improper skin care, and lifestyle habits such as smoking.

The most important factor is sun exposure which is your skin's worst enemy because it dries the skin and leads to the generation of free radicals that can damage skin cells. Research shows that 90% of what we think are signs of age are actually signs of over exposure to sunlight. Furthermore, approximately 70% of sun damage comes from everyday activities such as driving and walking to and from your car.

The ultraviolet-A rays that cause this enormous damage are present all day long in all seasons. These ultraviolet-A rays wear away the elasticity of the skin, causing wrinkling. The worst part is that the effects of the sun are cumulative, although they may not be noticeable for many years.

TIP: Did you know that natural beauty products are not always as advertised?

Manufacturers say that their products contain natural ingredients but the reality is that they contain tiny amounts compared to the artificial substances used. You find out by looking at the label of the product. The ingredients are listed in descending order, starting with the greatest amount contained. For example, a product may be labeled as rosemary, but the label shows only chemicals and artificial substances and not a drop of pure rosemary.

We recommend:

• Eat a balanced diet including fruits, vegetables, whole grain foods, seeds, nuts and legumes.

• Drink plenty of fluids every day. This help to keep the skin hydrated and flush away toxins.

• Obtain fatty acids from cold pressed vegetable oils.

• Avoid alcohol, caffeine and cigarettes. They dry the skin and encourage the development of wrinkles. Also the smoking habit uses the lips' muscles hundreds of times a day which contributes to wrinkling.

• Always protect your skin from the sun by applying a sunscreen with a sun protection factor (SPF) of at least 15 to all exposed areas of the skin.

• Avoid alcohol-based products. Use hazel or an herbal, floral water instead.

• Avoid using harsh soaps or solid cleansing creams. Use natural oils such as avocado oil to remove dirt and makeup.

• Do not apply heavy oils around the eye area before going to bed. Because it might cause the eye to be puffy in the morning.

• Take Vitamin E to protect against free radicals that can damage the skin and contribute to aging and wrinkles.

• Take Vitamin C to promote the formation of collagen, a protein that gives the skin flexibility. It also fights free radicals and strengthens the capillaries that feed the skin.

• Take Silica. It is important for skin strength and elasticity and also, stimulates collagen formation.

• Take Vitamin A. It is necessary for healing and the construction of new skin tissue.

• Take Vitamin B complex + Vitamin B12. They are anti stress and anti-aging vitamins.

• Take primrose or black currant seed oil. They are good healers for dermatitis, acne and others skin disorders.

• Use a collagen cream because it is very good for dry skin.

• Use elastin cream to help smooth existing wrinkles and prevent the appearance of new ones.

• To alleviate puffy eyes, peel a cucumber, cool it and place it in the eye area for 10 minutes. Repeat if necessary.

• To cleanse the pores, rub mush tomatoes over your face, then rinse.

• To protect your skin from free radical damage, add a few drops of green tea extract to your lotions or astringents.

• To moisture your skin, mash together grapes and honey, enough to make a paste, apply over your face as a mask. Leave it for 30 minutes then rinse away.

• To remove dead cells and improve skin texture, rub a small handful of dry short grain rice against your face for a couple of minutes.

- To soften and nourish the skin, mash half an avocado and apply over the face. Leave it on until it dries, then rinse with warm water.

Home Remedies For Allergies

An allergy is a hypersensitive reaction to a normally harmless substance. There are a variety of substances, termed allergens, that may trouble a sensitive individual.

Common allergens include pollen, animal dander, house dust, feathers, mites, chemicals, and a variety of foods. Some allergies primarily cause respiratory symptoms; others can cause such diverse symptoms as headache, fatigue, fever, diarrhea, stomachache, and vomiting. This entry addresses respiratory allergies, both chronic and seasonal (for a discussion of allergic reactions caused by foods. Home remedies for allergies can help reduce and treat allergies symptoms.

If you have allergies, you may suffer from a stuffy and/or runny nose, sneezing, itchy skin and eyes, and/or red, watery eyes. Needless to say, it can be very uncomfortable.

These symptoms occur because, in the presence of an allergen, the immune system releases chemicals called histamines to fight what it perceives as an invader. Home remedies for allergies can treat all of the above mentioned symptoms.

Histamines cause a string of reactions, including the swelling and congestion of nasal passages and increased mucus production. This is essentially a hypersensitive, or overactive, response by the body to an external stimulus. You will not suffer any of these side effect using this home remedies for allergies.

Whether allergies are seasonal or chronic depends on the particular allergen or allergens involved. Seasonal allergies tend to be caused by pollen. Ongoing or chronic allergies are usually caused by factors that are present in the environment year-round, such as animal dander, dust, or feathers. Chronic allergic rhinitis is a persistent inflammation of the mucous membrane lining the nasal passages that is caused by an allergic reaction. It is characterized by a stuffy, runny nose, frequent sneezing, and a tendency to breathe through the mouth. The eyes may be red and watery. Headache, itchiness, nosebleeds, and fatigue may be secondary complications. Dark circles under the eyes (called "allergic shiners"), along with a puffy look to the face, are frequently seen.

Home remedies for Allergies - Diet

Home remedies for allergies #1: ■ Drink lots of water to thin secretions and ease expectoration.

Home remedies for allergies #2: ■ If you have respiratory allergies, you may be allergic to certain foods. In addition to dairy products and wheat, common culprits include eggs, chocolate, nuts, seafood, and citrus fruits and juices. Try eliminating one of these foods for two weeks and watch for an improvement. Use an elimination or rotation diet to discover and work with food allergies.

Home remedies for allergies #3: Try eliminating dairy foods from your diet. Dairy

foods can thicken mucus and stimulate an increase in mucus production. If your

allergies are seasonal, it may also be helpful to avoid whole wheat during the allergy season; many allergy sufferers are sensitive to wheat.

Home remedies for allergies #4: Cut out cooked fats and oils. When your body is

under any type of stress, including the stress of an allergic reaction, the digestive system is not as strong as usual, and fats—which are difficult to digest at the best of times—can put a strain on the digestive system. Also, undigested fats contribute to mucus production and foster a toxic internal environment.

Home remedies for Allergies - Supplements

Home remedies for allergies #5: Calcium and magnesium are important nutrients for the allergy sufferer. They help to relax an over reactive nervous system. While symptoms are acute, take a supplement containing 750 to 1,000 milligrams of calcium and 500 milligrams of magnesium twice a day. Then take the same dosage once a day for two months.

Home remedies for allergies #6: Allergies are often related to the transformation and transportation of foods in the digestive system. Taking a digestive-enzyme supplement will enhance the assimilation and utilization of nutrients. Take a full-spectrum digestive-enzyme supplement providing 5,000 international units of lipase, 2,500 international units of amylase, and 300 international units of protease, plus 500 to 1,000 milligrams of pancreatin immediately after each meal.

Home remedies for allergies #7: Methylsulfonylmethane (MSM) is a good source of sulfur, a trace mineral that may help to reduce the severity of the allergic response. Take 500 milligrams three or four times daily, with meals.

Home remedies for allergies #8: Selenium is an antioxidant and works synergistically with vitamin E. Take 50 to 100 micrograms twice a day during the allergy season.

Home remedies for allergies #9: Vitamin C has anti-inflammatory properties. During acute flare-ups, take 1,000 milligrams five times a day for four to five days. Follow this with 1,000 milligrams three times a day for three weeks; then take 1,000 milligrams a day for two months. Some people with allergies find mineral absorb vitamin C or esterified vitamin C (Ester-C) easier to tolerate than simple ascorbic acid.

Home remedies for Allergies - Herbs

Home remedies for allergies #10: If your nasal mucus is green or yellow, you may have an infection on top of allergies. Take one dose of an echinacea and goldenseal combination formula supplying 250 to 500 milligrams of echinacea and 150 to 300 milligrams of goldenseal two to three times daily for five to seven days to help resolve the infection.

Home remedies for allergies #11: Nettle can be very helpful for drying out the sinuses.

It can be highly effective for chronic allergies. Take 150 to 500 milligrams two or three times daily, as needed, for two weeks.

Home remedies for allergies #12: Turmeric is an East Indian herb with natural anti-inflammatory properties. It is an excellent remedy for those who suffer from fatigue coupled with allergies. Take 500 milligrams three times daily.

Home Remedies For Headache

Virtually everyone gets a headache at one time or another. An estimated 17.6 percent of women and 6 percent of men in the United States experience headaches on more than an occasional basis, and some 20 million regularly experience cluster and migraine headaches. Home remedies are the best way to treat a headache because they are as common—and as difficult to cure—as the common cold and flu. Common causes of headache include stress; tension; anxiety; allergies; constipation; coffee consumption; eyestrain; hunger; sinus pressure; muscle tension; hormonal imbalances; temporomandibular joint (TMJ) syndrome; trauma to the head; nutritional deficiencies; the use of alcohol, drugs, or tobacco; fever; and exposure to irritants such as pollution, perfume, or after-shave lotions. Migraines result from a disturbance in the blood circulation in the head. (See MIGRAINE)

Headache experts estimate that about 90 percent of all headaches are tension headaches and 6 percent are migraines. Tension headaches, as the name implies, are caused by muscular tension. Another type of headache is the cluster headache. These are severe, recurring headaches that strike about 1 million Americans, and are widely considered to be the most painful type of headache.

Using home remedies for headaches is a great way to get rid of the pain without using drugs. Headaches can also be a sign of an underlying health problem. People who suffer from frequent headaches may be reacting to certain foods and food additives, such as wheat, chocolate, monosodium glutamate (MSG), sulfites (used in restaurants on salad bars), sugar, hot dogs, luncheon meats, dairy products, nuts, citric acid, fermented foods (cheeses, sour cream, yogurt), alcohol, vinegar, and/or marinated foods. Other possibilities to consider are anemia, bowel problems, brain disorders such as tumors, bruxism (tooth-grinding), hypertension (high blood pressure), hypoglycemia (low blood sugar), sinusitis, spinal misalignment, toxic overdoses of vitamin A, vitamin B deficiency, and diseases of the eye, nose, and throat. Dehydration also can cause headaches—often accompanied by a feeling of being flushed, a warm face, and a sense of heaviness in the head.

Unless otherwise specified, the dosages recommended here are for adults. For a child between the ages of twelve and seventeen, reduce the dose to three-quarters the recommended amount. For a child between six and twelve, use one-half the recommended dose, and for a child under the age of six, use one-quarter the recommended amount.

Home remedies for Headaches

Home remedies for headaches #1: Coenzyme Q10 plus Coenzyme A Improves tissue oxygenation. Take 30 mg twice daily.

Home remedies for headaches #2: Calcium and magnesium are Minerals that help to alleviate muscular tension. Use chelated forms.

Deficiency may be a cause of migraines. Relaxes muscles and blood vessels. Take 1,000 mg daily.

Home remedies for headaches #3: Glucosamine sulfate is a natural alternative to aspirin and other nonsteroidal anti- inflammatory drugs (NSAIDs).

Home remedies for headaches #4: Cayenne thins the blood, which reduces pain and allows beneficial blood flow.

Home remedies for headaches #5: Chamomile relaxes muscles and soothes tension.

Home remedies for headaches #6: Ginkgo biloba extract improves circulation to the brain, and may be helpful for certain types of headache.

Home remedies for headaches #7: Guarana can alleviate cluster headaches.

Home remedies for headaches #8: Use a homeopathic remedy suitable for the particular headache symptoms you are experiencing. Belladonna helps with sudden, severe pain that is worse on the right side, of the body. Natrum muriaticum is recommended for tension headaches and periodic headaches. Sanguinaria is good for pain that is sharp and splitting. Arsenicum album, kali bichrornium, Mecurius solubilis, and Pulsatilla all encourage drainage of the sinuses.

Home Remedies For Anxiety

Anxiety is the second most common psychological problem, yet remains undiagnosed 75% of the time. In our anxious age, doubts and fears can manifest as simple worries, free-floating anxiety, phobias (agoraphobia, social phobias, etc.), panic disorders and obsessive-compulsive tendencies. The latter may affect as many as 7 million Americans. Home remedies for anxiety offer the best approach to complement the traditional treatment.

Physical aspects of anxiety include stomach upsets, colitis, migraines, palpitations, hypertension and sweating. Anxiety after trauma, post traumatic stress syndrome (PTSD), is also increasingly common. Underlying, contributing factors are low blood sugar, food allergy, nutrient deficiency (fatty acids, B complex, etc.) and imbalances of the thyroid, ovaries or adrenals. Home remedies for anxiety can help you get this nutrient in.

Many of the herbs that help anxiety work on the same brain receptor sites as drugs like Valium, Xanax and Halcion. Herbs however, tend to be gentler, safer and non-addictive.

They have relaxant properties but also nourish and strengthen the nervous system. There are hundreds of home remedies for anxiety and nervous disorders.

Home remedies for Anxiety

Home remedies for Anxiety #1: California Poppy••—Eschscholtzia californica

• A tension-relieving, sedative, anti-anxiety and antispasmodic herb.

• Helps sleeplessness, quells headache and muscular spasm from stress.

• Gentle, non-addictive action that is safe for children and the elderly.

Home remedies for Anxiety #2: Chamomile•••—Matricaria recutita

• Tranquilizing effects, with action similar to drugs, i.e. Halcion, Valium.

• Reduces effects of stress-induced chemicals in the brain, while promoting healthy adrenal hormones (e.g. cortisol). Relieves pain and spasms.

• Aids digestion, cramping and back pain. Promotes restful sleep.

Home remedies for Anxiety #3: Hops••—Humulus lupulus

• Calms nerves, eases anxiety, restlessness and tension. For headaches from stress, insomnia / sleep loss, indigestion or effects of alcohol.

• Its sedative properties are not appropriate for use during depression.

Home remedies for Anxiety #4: Kava Kava•••—Piper methysticum

• Reduces anxiety, fear, tension; alleviates stress from many emotional, interpersonal and career factors. Improves performance; no grogginess.

• Relaxes muscles, relieves pain, insomnia and promotes restful sleep.

• Compares favorably to tranquilizers and benzodiazepines for anxiety.

Home remedies for Anxiety #5: Lemon Balrn•—Melissa officinalis

• Relaxing and tonic herb, reduces anxiety, restlessness and nervousness.

• Helps with panic disorder, palpitations, racing heart, overactive thyroid.

• For digestive upset from stress or anxiety; nausea, indigestion, colic.

• Anti-depressant. Good in synergistic combination with other herbs.

Home remedies for Anxiety #6: Linden••—Tilia europaea

• Reduces tension, promotes relaxation; mild mood-elevating qualities.

• Protects against illness due to stress, anxiety and overactive adrenal glands, including high blood pressure, palpitations, gastric ulcers.

Home remedies for Anxiety #7: Mothervvort••—Leonarus cardiaca

• A relaxing, tonic herb and mild sedative that gently relieves tension, anxiety when feeling under pressure. A heart, uterine and thyroid tonic.

• Relieves symptoms like a racing heart, shallow breathing.

Home remedies for Anxiety #8: Passionflower• •—Passiflora incarnata

• Sedative herb that relieves anxiety, tension, spasms, pains, neuralgia.

• Promotes restful, refreshed sleep; induces relaxation, mild euphoria.

• Gentle action, suitable for nervousness in children and the elderly.

Home remedies for Anxiety #9: Skullcap•••—Scutellaria laterifolia

• Relaxes, yet tones and renews the nervous system. Calms oversensitivity.

• Helps hysteria, depression and exhaustion, eases stress during PMS.

• Pain reliever and antispasmodic, decreases restlessness, nervousness.

Home remedies for Anxiety #10: St. John's Wort•••--Hypericum perfoliatum

• Effective long-term action for anxiety and tension, as well as irritability and depression. Also for mood changes during menopause and for pain syndromes, including fibromyalgia, arthritis and neuralgia.

Home remedies for Anxiety #11: Valerian• • •—Valeriana officinalis

• Sedative and muscle relaxant; for anxiety, stress, muscle tension and pain, nervous cramps, restlessness, insomnia, overwork or overstudy.

• For easing off drug dependency (both medical and recreational drugs).

• For after effects of chronic flu. Improves poor concentration.

Home remedies for Anxiety #12: Vervain••—Verbena officinalis

• Relaxing nervine; reduces tension, strengthens the nervous system.

• Reduces anxiety due to stress, PMS or menopause, calms hysteria.

• Useful for lingering depression after a cold or flu. Tones the liver.

Home remedies for Anxiety #13: Wild Lettuce•--Lactuca virosa

• Gentle tranquilizer, calming an overactive, excitable nervous system.

• Very suitable for anxious children or adolescents. Helps with insomnia.

• General pain reliever and antispasmodic, especially for irritable coughs.

Home remedies for Anxiety #14: Wood Betony••—Stachys officinalis

• Sedative action, relieves tension, anxiety and nervous exhaustion.

• Calms an overactive, edgy state. Relieves headaches and neuralgic pain.

• Strengthens neurological function and improves memory, clarity.

Home Remedies for Yeast Infection

Systemic infection with candida and other strains of yeast is epidemic today and is an underlying factor in many chronic conditions (e.g. migraines, colitis, obesity, fibromyalgia, chronic fatigue, sinusitis, PMS). This is a result of immune failure and contributes to immunity's progressive weakening. Home remedies for yeast infection can also be used in combination with other remedies for the above mention symptoms.

Other contributing causes include antibiotics, which destroy protective intestinal bacteria, and a variety of immune-damaging factors and environmental toxins. Sugar and carbohydrate excess, or estrogen imbalance (hormone therapy` pill, PMS), sweetens the tissues, creating a yeast breeding ground. Food allergies and a toxic digestive system (dysbiosis) complete the picture. Home remedies for yeast infection can reverse the imbalance and return it to normal levels.

Antifungal herbs must be used and alternated for some time. An integral part of treatment is yeast die-off or Herxheimer reaction, which can produce fatigue, headaches, digestive upset and so on. The side effects can be minimized by starting with low dosages, increasing gradually, and helping detoxification. A low-carb, high-protein diet, digestive enzymes, liver detoxification and immune-strengthening herbs are essential. Check below a list of home remedies for yeast infections. See also Candida

Home remedies for Yeast Infection

Home remedies for Yeast Infection #1: Black Walnut**—Juglans nigra

• Unripe, green hulls contain juglone, an effective antifungal agent.

• Assists with systemic candida, athlete's foot and ring worm infections.

• Also inhibits other fungi, cryptococcus, salmonella, staph, E. coli.

Home remedies for Yeast Infection #2: Cat's Claw* * *—Una de gato/Uncaria

tormentosa

• Has antimicrobial effects for fungi, viruses, bacteria, parasites.

• Important intestinal cleanser for dysbiosis, leaky gut, diverticulitis, colitis, Crohn's. Anti-aging, anti-inflammatory, immune strengthening.

Home remedies for Yeast Infection #3: Celandine*--Chelidonium majus

• Treats candida effectively; powerful liver detoxifier and hepatic strengthener; helps in removal of candida metabolites from the bloodstream.

Home remedies for Yeast Infection #4: Garlic***—Allium sativa

• Contains several antifungal ingredients; rapidly destroys yeast.

• Stimulates immune function. Highly antiseptic, effective in infections, and is beneficial for long-term use against chronic candida syndromes.

Home remedies for Yeast Infection #5: Goldenseal***—Hydrastis canadensis

• Strong antifungal effects, while healing intestinal mucus linings.

• Strengthens and detoxifies the liver; immune and white cell stimulant.

Home remedies for Yeast Infection #6: Yeast infection Tincture:

1 ounce tincture of black walnut husk (fresh)

1/2 ounce each tinctures lavender flowers, valerian root, pau d'arco.

10 drops tea tree oil.

Mix all the ingredients and shake well before each use. Take 2 to 3 dropperfuls a day.

Home Remedies for Fatigue Syndrome

Fatigue is the most common presenting complaint in doctor's offices, and can be part of scores of serious medical conditions, as much as from overwork or lack of sleep.

Underlying causes need to be identified, and natural medicine recognizes many less obvious contributing factors. These include chronic intestinal dysbiosis, liver overload, adrenal exhaustion, hidden infections (yeast, viral or parasitic) and food allergies.

Typical short-term solutions such as caffeine, tobacco, sugar and other stimulants are ultimately debilitating for the hormonal and nervous system. That is why home remedies for fatigue syndrome are the best long term option to compliment your treatment.

Herbal medicines should be directed toward the underlying causes, but for simple fatigue, tonic and adaptogenic herbs can be relied upon. These have the ability to increase vitality and well-being, balancing and improving the function of the body's major control systems—immune, hormonal, cardiovascular and nervous. Thus they are particularly suitable for the effects of prolonged stress, both physical and psychological.

This class of botanical medicines can help compensate for and overcome the effects of overwork, depression, prolonged illness and convalescence after illness. In this list of home remedies for fatigue syndrome you will find the whole spectrum of benefits.

Optimal effects occur when tonics are taken long term (i.e. one to six months). They are best taken in chronic illness, rather than acutely and are typically used in a cycle of 3 weeks on and one week off. See also Immune Weakness - Liver Conditions - Stress.

Home Remedies for Fatigue Syndrome

Home Remedies for Fatigue #1: Alfalfa**—Medicago sativa

• Improves appetite, digestion; produces mental clarity and well-being.

• Increases stamina and strength, augments ability to respond to stress.

• For convalescence after long illness, extreme stress. Reduces toxicity.

• High in phytoestrogens, stimulates the body's hormone production.

• Note that alfalfa sprouts and especially seeds are potentially toxic.

Home Remedies for Fatigue #2: Astragalus*** —Milk Vetch/Astragalus membranaceous

• For general weakness, fatigue, loss of appetite, shortness of breath.

• Adaptogenic herb that stimulates immune function, improves stamina.

335

- Anti-inflammatory, antiviral, antibacterial effects; good for flu, cold.

- Strengthens people with cancer, after radiation or chemotherapy.

Home Remedies for Fatigue #3: Cordyceps**—Cordyceps sinensis

- Builds strength, endurance, stamina and immunity. Reduces fatigue, promotes lung and kidney function. Increases blood flow to brain, heart.

- Increases male potency, female vitality. Improves appetite and sleep.

Home Remedies for Fatigue #4: Ginseng***—Panax Ginseng

- Strengthens adrenals, improves vitality and ability to handles stress.

- Improves physical and mental performance, stamina; enhances mood.

- Increases visual and motor coordination, increases work capacity.

- Antioxidant, inhibits formation of free radicals, stimulates immunity.

Home Remedies for Fatigue #5: Gotu Kola***—Centella asiatica

- Improves brain function, memory. Anti-stress, anti-anxiety, relaxant.

- Strengthens body's connective tissue and blood vessels, heals wounds.

- Tonic and rejuvenator, improves fertility, has anti-inflammatory effects.

Home Remedies for Fatigue #6: Licorice**—Glycyrrhiza glabra

• Provides steroid-like factors for the body's own production of adrenaline, cortisol; thus boosts adrenal function and adaptation to stress.

• Antiviral and immune-enhancing herb, valuable for weakened states.

Home Remedies for Fatigue #7: Maitake**—Grifola frondosa

• Immune-stimulating effects; increases activity of immune cells (killer cells, etc.), as well as immune-modulating chemicals (interleukin 2).

• D-fraction has shown positive results in Epstein-Barr and chronic fatigue; inhibits virus production, protects cells from attack by toxins.

Home Remedies for Fatigue #8: Oats***—Avena sativa

• Exhaustion from work, study, illness, drugs, alcohol, sexual excess.

• Nutritive effect on the brain, rather than temporary stimulatory effect.

• Greatly sharpens mental acuity, focus, memory before an exam etc..

• Eases heart palpitations, effective for insomnia due to over fatigue.

Home Remedies for Fatigue #9: Schisandra***—Schisandra chinensis

• Improves adrenal and nervous system capacity, counteracts effects of stimulants, coffee. Improves liver function and protects it from toxins.

• Increases work and efficiency level, improves mood, memory and sleep.

• Re-regulates immune system, helps skin problems, aphrodisiac effects.

Home Remedies for Fatigue #10: Siberian Ginseng***—Eleutherococcus senticosus

• Adaptogenic herb, excellent for exhaustion, fatigue, immune weakness.

• For effects of long stress (physical, emotional, mental) or after illness.

• Increases mental alertness, work output and athletic performance.

• Enhances adrenals, increases immunity and protects against toxins.

Home Remedies for Fatigue #11: St. John's Wort*—Hypericum perforatum

• Inhibits viral activity and replication of herpes virus and Epstein-Barr.

• Relieves depression that is a cause or effect of fatigue; improves sleep.

Home Remedies for Fatigue #12: Yerba Mate*—Ilex paraguariensis

• Stimulates like caffeine, but without causing nervousness; calms, balances the nervous system. Improves sleep and mood, reduces allergy.

• Antioxidant, increases oxygen to the heart and brain.

Home Remedies for Candida

The human body is normally host to a great variety of bacteria and fungi that play neutral or even helpful roles in normal bodily functions. A candida occurs when one of these organisms, the yeast Candida albicans, grows out of control. The resulting overgrowth is known as candidiasis. C. albicans only becomes a problem when the "good" bacteria that normally keep it in check, such as Lactobacillus acidophilus, become weakened. Candida infection may take the form of athlete's foot and jock itch.

Home remedies for candida is a great alternative.

Systemic candidiasis is an overgrowth of candida throughout the body. In the most severe cases, candida can travel throughout the body, causing a type of blood poisoning called candida septicemia.

Candidiasis affects both women and men. It is rarely transmitted sexually. It is most common in babies (an infected mother may pass it on to her newborn) and people with compromised immune systems. As it proliferates, the fungus releases toxins that further weaken the immune system. Home remedies for candida can also be used with remedies for the immune system.

Because candidiasis can affect many areas of the body at once, it can cause a variety of disorders and symptoms. In the mouth, C. albicans can produce thrush, or white plaques in the mouth and throat. In women, it is one of the sources of vaginitis, which produces itching, burning, and a sticky white or yellow discharge. Overgrowth of yeast may result in weak nails; skin infections, marked by redness, inflammation, and itching; or digestive upsets causing abdominal pain, constipation, diarrhea, heartburn, rectal irritation, and colitis. candidas may develop in the urethra or sinuses. Other symptoms can include fatigue, memory loss, mood swings, muscle and joint pain, nagging cough and congestion, and numbness or tingling in the fingers and toes. Home remedies for candida can help with many of these symptoms.

Additional symptoms can include diaper rash, kidney and bladder infections, canker sores, headaches, and depression. Candida may also be implicated in some cases of impotence and prostatitis.

The growth of C. albicans is spurred by several factors. Broad-spectrum antibiotics can kill off the good bacteria that keep the yeast under control. Home remedies for candida can be used with regular antibiotics.

Taking corticosteroid drugs has been linked to C. albicans overgrowth. C. albicans is a sugar-loving organism, so candidiasis can be aggravated by eating too much sugar, or by the high blood-sugar levels associated with diabetes. And yeast can overgrow if the immune system does not function as it should, especially in people with HIV infection or AIDS and other diseases that affect the immune system. An imbalance in PH levels in the body is also a likely cause. C. albicans overgrowth is also associated with chronic fatigue syndrome, and with chronic skin or vaginal irritation. Home remedies for candida reduce irritation and discomfort.

Conventional medicine uses various antifungal agents. Except for barberry and related herbs, which should not be used for more than two weeks at a time, it may be necessary to take herbs for as long as six months to control yeast overgrowth.

Home remedies for candida

Home remedies for Candida #1: Take Lactobacillus and bifidus probiotic supplements daily. These friendly bacteria grow to form a protective lining over the digestive tract that keeps yeast colonies from forming. Be sure to check expiration dates on the package. For vaginal infections, place the probiotic capsules in the vagina before going to bed every other night for two weeks.

Home remedies for Candida #2: Take 1,000 to 2,000 milligrams of caprylic acid daily with meals. This naturally occurring fatty acid is an effective antifungal for the treatment of candida. Since caprylic acid is readily absorbed by the intestines, it is necessary to take a timed-release or enteric-coated form so that the supplement is released gradually throughout the entire digestive tract.

Home remedies for Candida #1: Avoid refined sugar, honey, maple syrup, and fruit juices. Also avoid chewing gums flavored with xylitol, which may aggravate thrush.

· Avoid antibiotics, steroids, and birth control pills unless medically directed to take them.

Home remedies for Candida #3: Several different antifungal agents are used to treat yeast infections. Topical creams include butoconazole (Femstat 3) and miconazole (Monistat), some of which are now available without prescription. Nystatin (Mycolog, Mycostatin, Nilstat) is relatively safe because it is not absorbed from the gastrointestinal tract. Stronger agents include fluconazole (Diflucan), itraconazole (Sporanox), and ketoconazole (Nizoral). Use of ketoconazole should be avoided, if possible, since this drug can be toxic to the liver. If ketoconazole is called for, its use should be supervised by an infectious disease specialist.

Home remedies for Candida #4: If you take the prescription blood-thinner warfarin (Coumadin), you should consult your doctor before using over-the-counter vaginal miconazole products. Miconazole is an antifungal drug found in some creams and suppositories used to treat vaginal candida. Bleeding or bruising may occur if warfarin and vaginal miconazole are used together.

Home remedies for Candida #5: In otherwise healthy people, high sugar consumption has very little effect on the growth of yeast. Only when the balance of yeast and other naturally occurring bacteria is upset by antibiotic treatment or injury to the immune system does yeast overgrowth become a problem.

Home remedies for Candida #6: While yeast overgrowth in the mucous membranes lining the gastrointestinal tract, throat, nose, urethra, and vagina are relatively common, candidas of the blood and inner organs are extremely rare. The effects of candida on the endocrine, immune, and nervous systems are caused by changes in absorption of nutrients rather than by the candida itself.

Home remedies for Candida #7: If a breast-fed baby develops oral thrush or a nursing mother develops a thrush infection of the nipples, both the mother and the baby should be treated to eradicate the infection, even if only one of them seems to be affected.

Home Remedies for High Blood Pressure

Whether blood pressure is high, low, or normal depends on several factors: the output from the heart, the resistance to blood flow of the blood vessels, the volume of blood, and blood distribution to the various organs. All of these factors in turn can be affected by the activities of the nervous system and certain hormones. Home remedies for high blood pressure can treat many symptoms to help regulate blood pressure naturally.

If blood pressure is elevated, the heart must work harder to pump an adequate amount of blood to all the tissues of the body. Ultimately, the condition often leads to kidney failure, heart failure, and stroke. In addition, high blood pressure is often associated with coronary heart disease, arteriosclerosis, kidney disorders, obesity, diabetes, hyperthyroidism, and adrenal tumors. There are many great home remedies for high blood pressure in this site.

The list of circulatory disorders is almost endless and includes heart disease, strokes, hypertension, and atherosclerosis, to name a few. These and other circulatory conditions are the number-one cause of death in this country, killing nearly one million Americans every year. You could be a victim of this silent killer, make it a habit to use home remedies for high blood pressure to lower the risks.

As we age, our body's ability to keep a proper equilibrium between blood clotting and blood liquefaction begins to go awry. On the one hand, blood must clot if we are to keep from bleeding to death, yet, on the other hand, it must be free flowing and liquid in order to travel easily through the body's blood vessels. The older we get, the "stickier" our blood gets, and our blood's ability to flow diminishes. When this occurs, the stage is set for blood clots, clogged arteries, strokes, and heart attacks.

Warning signs associated with advanced hypertension may include headaches, sweating, rapid pulse, shortness of breath, dizziness, and visual disturbances.

Home remedies for high blood pressure

Home Remedies for High Blood Pressure #1:

Use cayenne (capsicum), chamomile, fennel, hawthorn berries, parsley, and rosemary for high blood pressure.

Caution: Do not use chamomile on an ongoing basis, as ragweed allergy may result.

Avoid it completely if you are allergic to ragweed.

Home Remedies for High Blood Pressure #2: Hops and valerian root are good for calming the nerves.

Home Remedies for High Blood Pressure #3: Drink 3 cups of suma tea daily.

Home Remedies for High Blood Pressure #4: Avoid the herbs ephedra (ma huang) and licorice, as these herbs can elevate blood pressure.

Home Remedies for High Blood Pressure #5: Follow a strict salt-free diet. This is essential for lowering blood pressure. Lowering your salt intake is not enough; eliminate all salt from your diet. Read labels carefully and avoid those food products that have "salt," "soda," "sodium," or the symbol "Na" on the label. Some foods and food additives that should be avoided on this diet include monosodium glutamate (Accent, MSG); baking soda; canned vegetables (unless marked sodium- or salt-free); commercially prepared foods; over-the-counter medications that contain ibuprofen (such as Advil or Nuprin); diet soft drinks; foods with mold inhibitors, preservatives, and/or sugar substitutes; meat tenderizers; softened water; and soy sauce.

Home Remedies for High Blood Pressure #6: Eat a high-fiber diet and take supplemental fiber. Oat bran is a good source of fiber.

Note: Always take supplemental fiber separately from other supplements and medications.

Home Remedies for High Blood Pressure #7: Eat plenty of fruits and vegetables, such as apples, asparagus, bananas, broccoli, cabbage, cantaloupe, eggplant, garlic, grapefruit, green leafy vegetables, melons, peas, prunes, raisins, squash, and sweet potatoes.

Home Remedies for High Blood Pressure #8: Include fresh "live" juices in the diet. The following juices are healthful: beet, carrot, celery, currant, cranberry, citrus fruit, parsley, spinach, and watermelon.

Home Remedies for High Blood Pressure #9: Eat grains like brown rice, buckwheat, millet, and oats.

Home Remedies for High Blood Pressure #10: Drink steam-distilled water only.

Home Remedies for High Blood Pressure #11: Take 2 tablespoons of flaxseed oil daily

CIRCULATORY TEA #1

- teaspoon burdock root

1 teaApoon goldenAeal root

- teaApoon cayenne

2 teaspoons slippery elm bark

2 AliceA ginger root

3 cups boiling water

Combine the above herbs in a nonmetallic container, and pour the boiling water over them. Steep for 3o minutes, cool, and strain. Take up to one cup a day, two tablespoons at a time.

CIRCULATORY TEA #2

2 teaspoons black cohosh root

4 teaspoons ginkgo biloba leaves cups boiling water

Combine the above herbs in a nonmetallic container, and pour the boiling water over them. Soak for 3o minutes, cool, and strain. Take two to three tablespoons at a time, up to six times a day.

Home Remedies for Nausea and Vomiting

Nausea is an unpleasant feeling that you are about to vomit. It is often accompanied by excess salivation and sometimes stomach cramping. A number of diseases and conditions can cause nausea, including food poisoning (and other bacterial infections), viral infections, overeating or overdrinking, gallstones, pancreatitis, and cancer. It can also occur because of motion sickness, headache, or pregnancy. There are some very powerful home remedies for nausea and vomiting.

Sometimes unpleasant smells or tastes, and even emotional anxiety, can bring on nausea.

In addition to those herbs listed below, other beneficial herbs to relieve nausea include bayberry, bee balm, chaparral, horehound, and Oregon grape. These are great herbs to make home remedies for nausea and vomiting.

Home remedies for nausea and vomiting

Home Remedies for nausea and vomiting #1:

NAUSEA TEA #1

1 teaspoon grated ginger root

1 teaspoon yerba mama root

1 teaspoon peppermint leaves

2 cups boiling water

Combine the above herbs in a nonmetallic container and cover with the boiling water; steep for 3o minutes; cool and strain. Take as needed, a tablespoon at a time up to two cups a day.

Home Remedies for nausea and vomiting #2: NAUSEA TEA #2

1 teaspoon catnip leaves

1 teaspoon chamomile flowers cup boiling water

Combine the above ingredients in a nonmetallic container and cover with the boiling water; steep for 2o to 3o minutes; cool and strain. Take as needed.

Home Remedies for nausea and vomiting #3: Cayenne***—Capsicum frutescens

• Anti-inflammatory; relieves nausea, vomiting, gas, indigestion.

• Promotes digestion, warms the stomach and stimulates appetite.

• Do not use in acute stages of inflammatory gastritis or stomach ulcer.

Home Remedies for nausea and vomiting #4: Chamomile***—Matricaria recutita

• Tranquilizing effects with action similar to drugs like Halcion, Valium.

• Reduces effects of stress-induced chemicals in the brain, while promoting healthy adrenal hormones (e.g. cortisol). Relieves pain, spasms.

• Also aids digestion, cramping, back pain. Promotes restful sleep.

Home Remedies for nausea and vomiting #5: Cinnamon*—Cinnamomum

zeylandicum

• Relieves nausea, vomiting. Treats gastroenteritis, stomach flu, diarrhea.

• Antibacterial, antiviral and antifungal; expels gas, reduces spasms.

• Warming, astringent and stimulating to the digestion, reduces mucus.

Home Remedies for nausea and vomiting #6: Cloves*—Eugenia caryophyllata

• Relieves nausea, prevents vomiting. Reduces gastrointestinal spasms.

• Expels gas, bloating; antibacterial and antiviral, eliminates parasites.

• A few drops of the oil or infusion may be taken for quick nausea relief.

Home Remedies for Hives Urticaria

Hives, called urticaria by the medical profession, is a skin condition that is characterized by sudden outbreaks of red, itchy welts on the skin. Any area of the body may be affected. The welts may vary in appearance, from tiny, goosebump-like spots to rashes that cover significant areas of the body. Hives usually go away within a few hours to two days, but in rare cases they become chronic and may last for six weeks or more.

Home remedies for hives urticaria can greatly reduce the time of the outbreak.

Many cases of hives are brought on as allergic reactions and coincide with the release of histamine in the body. The release of histamine into the skin produces an inflammatory reaction, with itching, swelling, and redness. Hives can cause significant discomfort, but it does not cause injury or damage to any vital organs. However, home remedies for hives urticaria help also improve the immune system.

The skin is the largest organ of the body. It is an important part of the excretory system.

The skin acts in conjunction with other systems in the body to remove toxins and waste.

Hives can be a natural reaction to the presence of a foreign substance in the body.

However, an offending substance need not enter the body to trigger an outbreak of hives. Home remedies for hives urticaria can treat the skin naturally.

Merely coming into contact with various substances, such as pesticides, soaps, shampoos, hair sprays, residues from laundry products or dry cleaning chemicals on clothing, or any other of a vast array of other seemingly innocuous household items can unleash a maddening attack of hives.

The severity of a hives outbreak can vary from case to case as well as from person to person. Some people can break out in hives if they merely touch a certain type of plant or bush; others may develop hives only with considerable exposure, such as overconsumption of a certain food. Chemicals are a major cause of hives for many people; anything from perfumes to household cleaners can trigger a reaction, as can nervous conditions, stress, certain foods, and alcohol.

Viruses also can cause hives. Hepatitis B and Epstein- Barr virus, the virus that causes infectious mononucleosis, are the two most common culprits. Some bacterial infections likewise can cause outbreaks of hives, both chronic and acute. An association between Candida albicans and chronic hives has been established in several clinical studies over the past twenty years.

Home remedies for Hives Urticaria

Home Remedies for Hives Urticaria #1:

Aloe**—Aloe vera

- Applied topically, reduces inflammation, provides protective coating.

- Cooling to the tissues, relieves itching, redness, stinging and pain.

- Internally, stimulates immunity and elimination of inflammatory toxins.

Home Remedies for Hives Urticaria #2: Bromelain***—Pineapple/Ananas comosus

- More effective anti-inflammatory than most drugs, decreases the allergic response, alleviating hives, skin irritations. Accelerates healing.

- Non-toxic in large internal doses; may be applied directly to the hives.

Home Remedies for Hives Urticaria #3: Burdock**—Arctium lappa

- A liver and blood detoxifier, diuretic, digestive stimulant; assists in clearance of cellular and lymphatic debris, reduces tissue swelling.

- Purifies skin problems such as hives, acne, boils, eczema and psoriasis

- Stimulates the immune system; antibacterial, antiviral, antifungal.

Home Remedies for Hives Urticaria #4:

Chinese Skullcap**—Scutellaria baicalensis

- Contains potent flavonoids that are anti-allergic and anti-inflammatory.

- Stabilizes body during increased immune stress or allergen overload.

- Cools conditions of "damp heat" such as hives, fever, infections.

Home Remedies for Hives Urticaria #5: Curcurnin***—Turmeric/Curcuma longa

- Stimulates the body's natural anti-inflammatory corticosteroids.

- Very effective natural antihistamine and antioxidant for hives and a variety of inflammatory skin ailments. Protects liver against toxins.

Home Remedies for Hives Urticaria #6: Echinacea* * *—Echinacea angustifolia

- Anti-inflammatory; reduces sensitivity to allergens, stings or bites.

- Encourages blood and lymph drainage, modulates and balances a hyper-reactive immune system, antiviral and antibacterial effects.

Home Remedies for Hives Urticaria #7: Ginger* * *—Zingiber officinale

- Rapidly quells the onset of hives, itching or other allergic responses.

- A potent anti-inflammatory and antihistamine, improves skin circulation, relieves swelling and carries away inflammatory waste products.

Home Remedies for Hives Urticaria #8: Goldenseal/Coptis/Oregon Grape**—

Berberis spp

• Soothing herbs for swelling, itching; ideal for hives and skin disorders such as boils, sores, abscesses and fluid-filled or pustular eruptions.

• Tonic and detoxifying to the liver, gall bladder, stomach and intestines.

Home Remedies for Hives Urticaria #9:

Green Tea***—Camellia sinensis

• Strong antihistamine, reducing hives and other allergic inflammations.

• High in antioxidant polyphenols and flavonoids that protects against oxidative, toxic damage to the tissues. Enhances the immune system.

Home Remedies for Hives Urticaria #10: Licorice**—Glycyrrhiza glabra

• Antihistamine and anti-inflammatory, increases levels of cortisone.

• Immune stimulating, improves stress response, antiviral activity.

• DGL form is not effective for allergy. Also use locally as a tea or lotion.

Home Remedies for Hives Urticaria #11: Nettles***—Urtica dioica

• Freeze-dried form provides fast-acting antihistamine, symptom relief.

• Anti-inflammatory and astringent to relieve swelling or edema of hives.

• Detoxifying and diuretic, encourages excretion of inflammatory wastes.

Home Remedies for Hives Urticaria #12: Quercetin***—Quercetin

• A non-toxic, potent antihistamine bioflavonoid, decreases inflammation of allergic skin and hay fever conditions. Strengthens capillaries

• May be taken acutely during hive outbreak or as a preventive measure.

Home Remedies for Hives Urticaria #13: Schisandra**—Schisandra chinensis

• Chinese herb that alleviates hives, eczema and swollen tissues.

• A tonic for the adrenals, increases ability to deal with chemical stress.

• Improves sluggish or deficient liver and protects it from various toxins.

Home Remedies for Hives Urticaria #14: Yarrow***—Achillea millefolium

• Pain-relieving astringent, antiseptic and anti-inflammatory action.

• Take internally or apply directly to hives to quell inflammation and pain associated with swollen tissues. Detoxifies tissues of cellular waste.

Home Remedies For Canker Sores

Canker Sores are painful small, craterlike ulcers. They are gray-based with red rims. They usually develop on the insides of the cheeks, the inner lips, and the loose parts of the gums, mouth, and lips. Less commonly, they can affect the esophagus and rest of the gastrointestinal tract. Home remedies for canker sores can help reduce pain and speed up healing.

There is usually a burning and tingling sensation starting twenty-four hours before the ulcers actually form, and it is most helpful to start treatment as soon as this is felt.

Canker sores can be so painful that they interfere with speaking, eating, and nutrition.

The best alternative for healing canker sores is to use home remedies.

If they are less than one centimeter (about one-half inch) in diameter, they are called minor aphthous ulcers. These usually heal by themselves within a week or two. If they are greater than 3 centimeters in diameter, they are classified as major aphthous ulcers, and it often takes six weeks for them to finally heal. When they do, they leave scars.

Both small and large ulcers often return, either singly or in crops.

Canker sores are the most common disorder to affect the oral mucous membranes, with between 20 and 50 percent of Americans affected. Women are more likely to be affected than men, usually starting in their twenties or thirties. Some people seem to have an inherited tendency to form canker sores. These people should always use home remedies to treat canker sores to avoid constant use of hash drugs.

Canker sores may be infectious, resulting from a local bacterial or viral infection. They commonly have one or more triggers, including food allergies, acidic mouth conditions, and minor injury to the tissues of the mouth, smoking, vitamin deficiencies, stress, extreme heat, fever, and premenstrual and postmenopausal hormonal changes. People with poorly functioning immune systems are also very susceptible to canker sores. Home remedies for canker sores can be used in combination with remedies for low immune system.

Home remedies for Canker Sores

Home remedies for canker sores #1: • Canker sores may be due to a deficiency of vitamin B12, folic acid, zinc, the amino acid lysine, or iron, so these nutrients may need to be supplemented aggressively. The following supplements are recommended for people with canker sores:

Home remedies for canker sores #2: • Vitamin B12. Take 1,000 micrograms daily.

Also take a vitamin-B complex with 100 milligrams of most of the major B vitamins three times a day, with meals.

Home remedies for canker sores #3: • Vitamin C with bioflavonoids. Take 1,000 milligrams three times a day, with meals.

Home remedies for canker sores #4: • Zinc. Take 50 to 100 milligrams a day.

Home remedies for canker sores #5: • Iron. Take 15 milligrams a day.

Home remedies for canker sores #6: • Folic acid. Take 400 milligrams twice a day.

Home remedies for canker sores #7: • L-Lysine. Take 4 grams (4,000 milligrams) daily for the first four days, and then cut back to 500 milligrams three times a day. Take this supplement on an empty stomach.

Home remedies for canker sores #8: Supplementation with acidophilus powder or capsules to restore the healthy balance of bacteria in the mucous membranes of the mouth is often helpful.

Home remedies for canker sores #9: • Applying the oil from one vitamin-E capsule directly to the sores helps to clear the lesions more quickly.

Home remedies for canker sores #10: Aloe vera juice, available by the gallon, swished around in your mouth three times a day like a mouthwash, often yields good results. Aloe contains salicylates, which are anti-inflammatory and relieve pain, and it also has mild antibacterial properties.

Home remedies for canker sores #11: Chlorophyll is a blood detoxifier. Chlorophyll tablets are sometimes chewed for the treatment of canker sores.

Home remedies for canker sores #12: A soothing antiseptic mouth rinse can be made of 1/2 teaspoon of goldenseal powder and 1/4 teaspoon salt dissolved in 1 cup of warm water. Use this as a mouth rinse four times a day. Goldenseal helps reduce inflammation of mucous membranes, and has also been shown to have antibacterial properties.

Home Remedies For Boils

A boil or furuncle is a bacterial infection with pus that develops around a hair follicle.

Boils are very contagious and potentially serious if the infection spreads. A boil starts out as a tender, red, hot, tense bump and develops a yellowish point within 2 to 4 days.

Boils are very painful, especially if they occur in skin that cannot move freely. The boil can burst open, discharging pus but relieving some of the pain. There are many home remedies for boils that can reduce the symptoms.

Unfortunately, boils heal with scarring.

Boils usually occur in areas that are hairy or that are exposed to lots of movement and friction. These include areas under the belt and on the neck, face, scalp, underarms, and buttocks. Boils can become chronic and come back time and again in the same areas.

Our home remedies for boils reduce the risk of developing chronic boils.

The most common bacteria found in boils is Staphylococcus aureus (staph bacteria).

They may be caused by other types of bacteria, however, depending on the location of the boil and the individual's immune function. In rare cases, boils may be a sign of an underlying immune problem or other disease. People with diabetes, alcoholism, cancer, or HIV/AIDS, and those on chemotherapy are especially susceptible to developing boils. Please use these home remedies for boils.

Home remedies for boils

Home remedies for boils #1:

• Vitamin A. Take 25,000 international units daily for two weeks.

Home remedies for boils #2:

• Beta-carotene. Take 25,000 international units daily for two weeks.

Home remedies for boils #3:

• B-complex vitamins. Take a balanced B-complex supplement daily

Home remedies for boils #4:

• Vitamin C with bioflavonoids. Take 3,000 milligrams daily.

Home remedies for boils #5:

• Zinc. Take 50 milligrams daily for two weeks.

Home remedies for boils #6:

• Astralagus tea helps to enhance immunity. Drink eight glasses a day.

Home remedies for boils #7: Calendula ointment can to applied to the skin overlying an unbroken boil to decrease inflammation and act as an antiseptic. Is Garlic is a natural antibiotic and immune-system booster. It can be taken in capsule form.

Home remedies for boils #8: • Goldenseal-root powder can be mixed with enough boiling water to make a paste and used as a topical poultice to draw out the boil.

Home remedies for boils #9: A mixture of 25 grams (2,500 milligrams) of powdered slippery elm, 3 drops of eucalyptus oil, and just enough boiling water to form a thick paste can be applied to the boil. Leave it on until the paste cools, then make a fresh batch and reapply it. Repeat this until the pus is discharged from the boil. Marshmallow leaf or figwort can also be made into a poultice to draw out pus.

Home remedies for boils #10: Tea tree oil can be applied externally to a boil as an antiseptic against bacteria and fungi. The pure oil will probably irritate inflamed skin, but a mixture of a few drops in a couple of tablespoons of any vegetable oil should not cause a problem. Do not take tea tree oil internally.

Home remedies for boils #11: • A tea made from two parts wild indigo to one part each of echinacea, pasque flower, and poke root can be drunk three times a day to speed healing. The tea can also be applied externally to a boil to limit infection.

Home Remedies for Body Odor

Unpleasant body odor, or bromhidrosis, is most frequently due to excessive perspiration from the eccrine or apocrine sweat glands. This in turn causes an overgrowth of bacteria on the skin. The bacteria break down the top layer of skin cells and the sweat, forming chemicals that produce the unpleasant smell. Home remedies for body odor can control bacteria.

Apocrine bromhidrosis rarely occurs before puberty, since the apocrine sweat glands virtually do not function before then. As most apocrine sweat glands are located in the armpits, this is the smelliest area. Home remedies for body odor can help you make your own natural deodorant.

People in groups that tend to have larger numbers of apocrine sweat glands, such as people of African ancestry, are affected to a greater extent than those who tend to have fewer apocrine sweat glands, such as older adults and people of Asian descent. Poor hygiene, of course, is another reason unpleasant smells come off the body. Diet can also be a factor.

Sweat containing high levels of garlic, curry, or other spices also has a repellent odor.

Taking certain medications can cause bad body odor, too.

Excessive eccrine sweating of the feet, most common in young men, is another common cause of bad body odor. Bromhidrosis from the feet occurs when the thick, warm, sodden skin becomes a breeding ground for numerous bacteria. Eccrine bromhidrosis can also occur in areas where skin contacts skin, especially between the thighs. This can be made worse by obesity and diabetes. Using home remedies for body odor can help reduce foot odor.

Other, more serious causes of offensive body odor include nutrient deficiencies, such as zinc deficiency; underlying medical problems such as genetic metabolic disorders, liver disease, or diabetes; and gastrointestinal problems such as parasites or chronic constipation. You should seek your physician's expertise to screen for these problems if excessive sweating, poor hygiene, or a spicy diet are not factors in causing the unpleasant body odor.

Home remedies for body odor

Home Remedies for body odor #1:

NUTRITIONAL SUPPLEMENT'S FOR BODY ODOR:

• The following supplements have been found to be helpful for body odor:

• Vitamin A. Take 25,000 international units daily for two weeks.

• Vitamin-B complex. Take a supplement containing 100 milligrams of each of the major B vitamins daily Also take an additional 50 milligrams of vitamin B6 (pyridoxine) daily and 50 milligrams of vitamin B1 (thiamine) twice a day while the problem exists, then cut back to 20 milligrams every other day for three weeks.

• Vitamin C. Take 3,000 milligrams daily

• Zinc. Take 50 milligrams daily.

Home Remedies for body odor #2:

HERBAL TREATMENT FOR BODY ODOR:

Alfalfa tablets contain a lot of chlorophyll, which has a deodorizing effect.

• Chlorophyll, available in soft gel capsules and chewable tablets, helps reduce

embarrassing body odors.

• Parsley also is a good source of chlorophyll. Munching on several sprigs of parsley a day can help with body odor.

Home Remedies for body odor #3:

NATURAL DEODORANT FOR BODY ODOR:

• Make an herbal spray deodorant by combining 5 drops each of sage, coriander, and lavender essential oils with 2 ounces of distilled witch hazel. Shake before each use.

Home Remedies for Psoriasis

Psoriasis is among the most common and most difficult to control of all skin diseases, affecting about 2 percent of the population. It affects men and women equally, and usually appears between the ages of fifteen and thirty. It generally follows a chronic course of acute flare-ups alternating with periods of remission.

The word psoriasis is derived from the Greek psora, which means "to itch." Salmon-red bumps with a silvery scale appear on the skin, get bigger, and grow together to form large plaques. Lesions of psoriasis vary in size from fractions of an inch in diameter to large plaques covering most of the body and requiring hospitalization. Places on the body most commonly affected by psoriasis include the elbows, knees, scalp, and sacral areas. The nails are involved in about one-half of cases, with pitting, breaking, thickening under the nail, or thickening of the nail itself. In addition, between 10 and 30 percent of people with psoriasis also suffer from psoriatic arthritis, which can be quite painful.

Because of the chronic, difficult nature of psoriasis, professional help is needed in all but the least severe cases.

There appear to be many reasons why some people develop psoriasis and others do not.

It has a tendency to be inherited—about one-third of those who have it have another family member with psoriasis. Several studies have documented the relationship between specific stresses and the start and flare-ups of psoriasis. Almost half of all people with psoriasis report that a specific stressful event occurred within one month before the first episode of psoriasis.

Home remedies for Psoriasis

Home remedies for Psoriasis #1: Herbal liver tonics, together with tissue and blood cleansers, or alternatives, form the most important initial part of herbal treatment for psoriasis. Slightly less important are nerve tonics, or nervines, which soothe the nerves and lessen the itching of psoriasis.

Home remedies for Psoriasis #2: Applying aloe vera gel to the lesions can help. Dr. Andrew Weil reported that 83 percent of psoriasis patients who applied aloe-vera cream three times a day for up to four weeks noted an improvement. Dr. Weil recommends using pure aloe vera gel instead of an aloe vera cream that contains other ingredients.

Home remedies for Psoriasis #3: Apple-cider vinegar diluted in water can be used to temporarily help relieve itching and scaling. Apple cider vinegar or white vinegar can also be diluted in three to four times as much lukewarm water and poured over the head, rubbed in, left for one minute, and then rinsed out. Or you can add 1/2 cup of cider vinegar to a tubful of bath water to help restore acidity to the skin.

Home remedies for Psoriasis #4: Banana peel is a key ingredient in Exorex. This is a lotion concocted from coal tar and a specific essential fatty acid from banana peel that is associated with the immune system. Reportedly, the idea was derived from Zulu folklore, in which banana peels have been used for a variety of skin ailments for years.

Home remedies for Psoriasis #5: Burdock root can help improve flare-ups of psoriasis.

Take 20 to 40 drops of tincture three times a day.

Home remedies for Psoriasis #6: Chamomile is widely used in Europe for treating psoriasis. It contains anti-inflammatory flavonoid compounds. If you have ragweed allergies, however, do not use chamomile, as it is a member of the ragweed family.

Home remedies for Psoriasis #7: Castor oil is particularly helpful when left overnight on thick, small, well-circumscribed lesions. If cold-pressed castor oil is mixed with baking soda, it has been found to greatly improve thick, scaly heel skin, as long as the skin isn't cracked.

Home remedies for Psoriasis #8: Cayenne pepper has anti-inflammatory properties and helps with healing. Two clinical trials reviewed in the November 1998 issue of Archives of Dermatology reported that 0.025 percent capsaicin cream, made from hot peppers, works to reduce the redness and scaling in psoriasis. Capsaicin cream is available over the counter as Capzasin-P or Zostrix. It should be used over a six-week period. Care should be taken not to apply it to broken skin.

Home remedies for Psoriasis #9: Common figwort helps to clear psoriatic plaques.

The recommended dose is 2 milliliters of tincture, taken twice a day.

Home remedies for Psoriasis #10: Dandelion tincture is useful for stimulating bile flow and clearing toxins out of the system. It is frequently combined with yellow dock (see below) for this purpose. The recommended dose is 30 to 60 drops twice a day.

Home remedies for Psoriasis #11: Echinacea tincture is occasionally used for psoriasis. It boosts the immune system, and so may decrease the incidence of colds, which can lead to flare-ups in some individuals. The recommended dose is 20 to 30 drops three times a day for up to ten days. Stop for two weeks, then repeat.

Home remedies for Psoriasis #12: Emu oil contains essential fatty acids and may be helpful for psoriasis. Apply it to the lesions as directed by the manufacturer.

Home remedies for Psoriasis #13: Flaxseed oil is chemically similar to fish oil and helps treat psoriasis. Adding flaxseed oil to salad dressing is a good way to get this helpful supplement into your diet. Take 1%2 tablespoons of flaxseed oil daily.

Home remedies for Psoriasis #14: Fumitory contains fumaric acid, which has been found to be very helpful for psoriasis. Make a strong tea from fumitory and apply it to the affected areas with a cotton ball twice a day.

Home remedies for Psoriasis #15: Garlic is detoxifying and includes a number of sulfur-containing compounds. Sulfur deficiency may contribute to psoriasis. Take three to six garlic capsules daily.

Home remedies for Psoriasis #16: Goldenseal tincture helps to clear the body of toxins that lead to flareups. Take 20 to 30 drops twice a day for up to ten days at a time.

Home remedies for Psoriasis #17: Gotu kola extract reduces inflammation and speeds skin healing. In India, it has been used for psoriasis for hundreds of years. Take 200 milligrams three times a day for one month.

Home remedies for Psoriasis #18: Liquid licorice extract, applied directly to the affected areas with a cotton ball, is felt by some naturopaths to work as well as corticosteroid creams.

Home remedies for Psoriasis #19: Flaxseed oil, applied to affected areas twice a day, is said to help heal psoriasis. Avocado, garlic, and walnut oils, applied topically twice a day to the psoriatic patches, are equally helpful for moisturizing and healing.

Home remedies for Psoriasis #20: Milk thistle cleanses and protects the liver, increases bile flow, and helps in blood purification. It also helps to correct the abnormal cell replication present in psoriasis. Take 300 milligrams of milk-thistle extract three times a day.

Home remedies for Psoriasis #21: Neem-seed oil, an Ayurvedic herbal remedy, is highly recommended by some psoriasis sufferers. It was introduced to the United States in 1994 from India and Pakistan. Neem lotions are usually found in East Indian markets.

Home Remedies for Itching

Itching is a superficial sensation in the skin, probably originating at the border between the epidermis and the dermis. Histamine, a body chemical released in response to contact with an irritant of some kind, is thought to be one of the most common triggers for itching, although there are other chemical mediators in the skin and blood.

There are many causes of itching. Common causes of acute itching include allergies to plants, pollens, cats, dogs, feathers, perfumes, cosmetics, cleaning solutions, other chemicals, and smoke. Short-lived skin problems such as very dry skin, fungal infection, lice, scabies, and sunburn are also frequent reasons for itching. Pregnancy can sometimes produce itching and related skin problems.

Home remedies for Itching

Home remedies for Itching #1: A paste made from aloe vera gel and green clay soothes the skin.

Home remedies for Itching #2: Chamomile cream, calendula lotion, or comfrey ointment can be applied directly to the itchy areas as often as needed. They have anti-inflammatory properties that help to relieve your discomfort.

Home remedies for Itching #3: Jewelweed, otherwise known as impatiens, can be boiled in a gallon of water, strained and cooled. The liquid stops itching extremely well.

In fact, in clinical trials, it worked just as well as prescription cortisone creams.

Jewelweed is a perennial wildflower that should be available at herb shops and through herbalists. It is not the same plant as the flowering annual called impatiens that is commonly sold in nurseries and garden centers.

Home remedies for Itching #4: An herbal tea made from two parts each of agrimony and chamomile and one part each of stinging nettle and heart's-ease can be taken three times a day as an aid to soothing the itching. In addition to drinking the tea, dip a clean cloth into it and apply it as a compress to the affected areas for five minutes every half hour, as needed. Other plants containing naturally antihistaminic compounds from which you can make a combination tea include basil, fennel, ginkgo, oregano, tarragon, tea, thyme, and yarrow. These teas should be used to compress the affected areas of itchy skin, as well as drunk three times a day

Home remedies for Itching #5: Diluted chamomile, lavender, and rosemary essential oils are soothing and relaxing, and help ease itching. You can add up to 10 drops of any of these oils (or a combination) to a tubful of water to make an aromatherapy bath, or you can dilute them in a carrier oil such as jojoba oil and apply it to the hives with a compress.

Home remedies for Itching #6: Rhus toxicodendron 30x or 15c is recommended for itching, especially if it is accompanied by joint pain or fever, or if discomfort is worse with the cold or scratching. Take one dose four times a day, up to a total of eight doses.

Home Remedies for Rash

An inflammation of the skin is used to describe many different types of rashes. The skin may itch, flake, scale, thicken, ooze, crust, and/or redden, depending on the type of dermatitis. Rashes can develop anywhere on the body. Certain locations are typical for different forms of rashes.

Atopic dermatitis, or eczema, the "itch that rashes" is a chronic, common problem that affects many people and for which there are many possible therapies. It is discussed in its own section (see Eczema). Contact dermatitis is probably the most common type of dermatitis. It is caused by irritation or allergy to something the skin comes in contact with. Types of rashes include irritant contact dermatitis, allergic contact dermatitis, and photoallergic contact dermatitis. A common type of allergic contact dermatitis is the rash of poison ivy, oak, and sumac. These also are described in their own section (see Poison Ivy, Oak, and Sumac).

Seborrhea (seborrheic dermatitis) is another distinct type of rash, and is discussed in its own section as well.

Home remedies for Rash

Home remedies for Rash #1: • Naturopaths believe that when waste products build up and exceed the capacity of the liver and kidneys to get rid of them, the skin has to eliminate the wastes. This can result in dermatitis. The following herbs cause sweating, which naturopaths feel is a good way to excrete the toxins that are trying to get out of your body:

Home remedies for Rash #2: Burdock root. Take 500 milligrams three times a day, with meals.

Home remedies for Rash #3: Sarsaprilla root. Take it as directed by the manufacturer.

Home remedies for Rash #4: Yarrow. Take it as directed by the manufacturer.

Naturopaths recommend one or more of the follow blood cleansers for rash:

Home remedies for Rash #5: Chaparral root. Take it as directed by the manufacturer.

Home remedies for Rash #6: Dandelion root. Take it as directed by the manufacturer.

Home remedies for Rash #7: Echinacea. Take it as directed by the manufacturer.

Home remedies for Rash #8: Goldenseal. Take 500 milligrams three times a day, with meals.

Home remedies for Rash #9: Pau d'arco. Take 500 milligrams three times a day, with meals.

Home remedies for Rash #10: Poke root. Make a tea by steeping 1 tablespoon of the herb in a cup of water. Drink this twice a day.

Home remedies for Rash #11: Red clover. Take 500 milligrams three times a day.

Home remedies for Rash #12: Yellow dock root. Take it as directed by the manufacturer.

Home remedies for Rash #13: The appropriate specific herbal therapy depends on the cause, location, and type of rash. However, the following therapies will all help relieve itching, no matter what sort of dermatitis you have:

Home remedies for Rash #14: Aloe vera gel and green clay soothe the skin.

Home remedies for Rash #15: Chamomile cream, calendula lotion, or comfrey ointment should be applied directly to the itchy areas as often as needed, as their anti-inflammatory properties will help relieve your discomfort.

Home remedies for Rash #16: Chickweed infusion can be used to bathe the area to stop itching.

Home remedies for Rash #17: Cucumber puree, made from peeled, blended fresh cucumbers, can be applied directly to the affected area for three minutes to relieve your itching and pain.

Home remedies for Rash #18: Jewelweed, also known as impatiens, can be boiled in a gallon of water, strained, and cooled. The liquid stops itching extremely well. In fact, in clinical trials, it has worked just as well as prescription cortisone creams. Note that while it is sometimes called impatiens, jewelweed is not the same plant that is sold as a flowering annual in home and garden centers.

Home remedies for Rash #19: An herbal tea made from two parts each of agrimony and chamomile and one part each of stinging nettle and heart's-ease can be taken three times a day as an aid to soothing the itching. In addition to drinking the tea, dip a clean cloth into it and apply it as a compress to the affected areas for five minutes every half hour, as needed. Other plants containing natural antihistaminic compounds from which you can make a combination tea include basil, fennel, ginkgo, oregano, tarragon, tea, thyme, and yarrow. These teas should be used in compresses applied to the itchy areas, as well as drunk three times a day.

Anti-Aging Remedies

Life span is ultimately determined by the fact that cells can only replicate a certain number of times—a genetically predetermined cut-off point that prevents physical immortality. Understanding this, most researchers still believe that humans should live 120 years or more. Why then is the average life span hovering around age 70? We deteriorate mainly due to damage from free radicals, produced as a byproduct of normal metabolism, or created by various toxins, pollutants, allergens, heavy metals, etc.

Additionally, 75% of Americans are not getting enough free radical fighting antioxidants, such as vitamin E, selenium or even vitamin C. These are quickly used up under stress, while hormonal, immune and neurological imbalances further accelerate aging.

A number of herbs are highly prized and renowned for their anti-aging and longevity-promoting effects. Science has extensively verified that these complex plant medicines have the definite ability to prolong the duration and quality of life. Many of these anti-aging herbs are adaptogens and tonics, normalizing metabolic, hormonal and neurological systems and stimulating cellular regeneration. Others have more focused effects on the brain, heart or immunity. They are safe for long-term use and disease prevention. See also Immune Weakness - Memory - Stress.

Anti-Aging Remedies

Anti-Aging Remedies #1: Ashwaganda***—Withania somnifera

• Tonic that slows aging rejuvenates tissues throughout the body.

• Clears the mind, strengthens the nerves, promotes restful sleep.

• Improves memory, cholesterol, sexual ability; lessens hair graying.

Anti-Aging Remedies #2: Fo-Ti***—Polygonum multiflorum

• Chinese tonic herb that promotes longevity, strengthens the blood, improves vitality, sexual vigor and fertility and can reduce hair graying.

• Lowers cholesterol, improves arteriosclerosis, and regulates blood sugar.

Anti-Aging Remedies #3: Garlic**—Allium sativa

• Protects nervous system, improves brain function, memory, learning.

• Prevents/treats arteriosclerosis, reduces clotting, lowers cholesterol.

• Increases life span in animal tests; inhibits viruses, bacteria, parasites.

Anti-Aging Remedies #4: Ginseng* * *—Panax ginseng

• Rejuvenating, stimulating adaptogen, yet helps calm nerves, increases vitality; reduces

exhaustion; increases stamina, speeds wound healing.

• Enhances immune system; balances metabolism and stress response.

Anti-Aging Remedies #5: Gotu Kola***—Centella asiatica

• Rejuvenating, longevity herb in the Ayurvedic and Chinese traditions.

• Increases intelligence, memory, creativity, learning ability, reduces mental fatigue.

Strengthens nervous system, adrenals and immune system.

• Improves wound healing, reduces scar tissue, and increases circulation.

Anti-Aging Remedies #6: Green Tea**—Camellia sinensis

• High in vitamins, minerals, antioxidants and flavonoids and especially polyphenols;

decreases cellular and tissue damage incurred with aging.

• Protective against cancer, heart diseases and is an immune stimulant.

Anti-Aging Remedies #7: Hawthorn**—Crataegus oxycantha

• Heart and circulation tonic; normalizes blood pressure, heart rhythm.

• Slows aging process, protects connective tissue and blood vessel walls.

• Reduces atherosclerosis, helps adaptation to physical and mental stress, protects

against radiation, improves digestion and assimilation.

Anti-Aging Remedies #8: Licorice**—Glycyrrhiza glabra

• Traditional Chinese longevity herb; stimulates adrenal glands, balances

and conserves cortisol and energy during stress. Anti-inflammatory.

• Has potent antioxidants that protect the digestive tract, liver and other tissues from the damaging effects of aging. Inhibits atrophy of thymus.

Anti-Aging Remedies #9: Maca**—Lepidium meyenii

• Ancient Peruvian herb that increases vitality, strength and stamina.

• Invigorates libido and is a sexual restorative in both men and women.

• Alleviates signs of decreasing hormones in middle age and menopause.

Anti-Aging Remedies #10: Reishi***—Ganoderma lucida

• A traditional "elixir of immortality" in Traditional Chinese Medicine.

• Treats a wide range of conditions, including heart disease and cancer.

• Normalizes blood pressure, cholesterol, platelet stickiness. Enhances immune and liver health, helps indigestion, eases tension, improves sleep.

Anti-Aging Remedies #11: Rhodiola**—Golden Root/Rhodiola rosea

• Increases immunity, prolongs life span, increases exercise capacity.

• Clears toxins, strengthens nervous and digestive system. Reduces fatigue.

Anti-Aging Remedies #12: Siberian Ginseng**—Eleuthrococcus senticosus

• Called the "king of adaptogens," has a wide range of vitalizing effects.

• Increases hearing, improves eyesight, supports immunity and stress adaptation.

Increases mental and physical work capacity.

Anti-Aging Remedies #13: Suma**—Pfaffia paniculata

• An adaptogen that is antiviral, antibacterial and immune stimulating.

• Increases muscle mass, protein production, overall physical endurance.

• Balances hormones, reduces blood sugar, cholesterol, triglycerides.

• Reduces fatigue, promotes liver and kidney regeneration, skin healing.

Home Remedies For backache

Backache affects at least 80% of people at some time, and most often concentrates in the low back. Poor postural habits are a major contributing cause, while other factors include repeated strains or microtrauma, muscle tension, nutritional deficiencies and reflex irritation from related internal organs. When repeated episodes of injury are added to this mix, the discs become subject to thinning, deterioration or rupture. These events can also gradually lead to arthritic changes.

With nerves close by, swelling or compression in the spine often results in neuritis, lumbar neuralgia or sciatica.

Herbal medicines are used similarly to medical drugs in this type of condition, though with far more safety. Both the anti-inflammatory and pain-relieving qualities of plants can be used effectively and taken for prolonged periods of time. Other benefits are relief of muscle spasm and repair of connective tissue and cartilage tissue. Bioflavonoids and other healing factors contained in herbs, along with well-known nutritional substances like glucosamine sulphate, can complete deeper repair and strengthening of tissues.

The herbs listed under Arthritis can provide further help for chronic joint dysfunction. If nerves become inflamed or compressed, additional sedative and nerve-repairing herbs may be needed. See also Arthritis

Use These Home Remedies for backache

Home Remedies for backache #1: Barberry* *—Berberis vulgaris

• For low backache, often related to kidney weakness or congestion.

• For sciatica and neuralgia with radiating pain and weakened muscles

• Use in rheumatic disorders, sciatica, bursitis, neuralgia and gout.

Home Remedies for backache #2: Black Cohosh**—Cimicifuga racemosa

• Anti-inflammatory effects, relaxing muscle spasms in low back and neck.

• Suitable for wry neck (torticollis), sciatica, neuralgia and intercostal (rib) neuralgia. Treats muscle pain associated with fibromyalgia, arthritis.

Home Remedies for backache #3: Black Haw***—Viburnum prunifolia

• With aspirin-like ingredients, relieves spasms and neuralgia of back and neck, sciatica, leg cramps, tension headache, wry neck, digestive spasm.

• A nervous system tonic and sedative, helps backache during menses.

Home Remedies for backache #4: Boswellia***—Boswellia serrata

• Strong anti-inflammatory effects, reduces stiffness and pain.

• Works for acute problems, but needs 2-4 weeks for maximal effects.

• Improves circulation around inflamed joints, ligaments, tendons.

Home Remedies for backache #5: Bromelain**—Pineapple/Ananas comosus

• Enzyme found in pineapple stem, helps resolve late stages of inflammation, speeding healing and reducing the potential for scar tissue.

Home Remedies for backache #6: Corydalis*—Corydalis soldida

• Chinese herb that relieves pain of all kinds, especially from injury.

• Sedative, analgesic, relives spasm and abdominal pain, dysmenorrhea.

• Often used in combination with other complementary herbs.

Home Remedies for backache #7: Devil's Claw**—Harpagophytum procumbens

• Anti-inflammatory and pain-relieving herb, with rapid results.

• Useful for low backache, arthritis and chronic rheumatic disorders, neuralgia and headaches. The whole herb preparation works best.

Home Remedies for backache #8: Dong Quai**—Angelica sinensis

• Reported to possess 1.5 times the analgesic activity of aspirin.

• Relieves backache, cramping, muscular spasms and inflammation.

• Also for menstrual cycle regulation, anemia; a liver and heart tonic.

Home Remedies for backache #9: Horse Chestnut*—Aesculus hippocastanum

• Low back, sacrum, and sacroiliac pain. Stiff, weak back that "gives out."

• Helps with arthritic and rheumatic backache with heaviness, swelling.

Home Remedies for backache #10: Jamaican Dogwood***—Piscidia erythrina

• Strong sedative, pain-relieving and antispasmodic effects.

• Especially valuable for muscular back spasms and pain, but also used in asthma, menstrual pain, insomnia, toothache or nervous conditions.

Home Remedies for backache #11: Kava Kava**—Piper methysticum

• Relaxes muscles, reduces internal and external spasms and cramps.

• Pain reliever, plus enhances pain-reducing effects of aspirin and drugs.

• No hangover, tolerance, build-up or addiction, typical of medical drugs.

Home Remedies for backache #12: Meadowsweet*—Filipendula ulmaria

• Herbal forerunner of aspirin provides anti-inflammatory pain relief.

• No gastric irritation like medical NSAIDs; neutralizes stomach acids and general internal acidity.

Home Remedies for backache #13: Valerian**—Valeriana officinalis

• Relaxing and sedative effects, reduces transmission of pain signals.

• Muscle relaxant, relieves muscle spasms and contractures due to stress and tension; eases menstrual pain, colic, asthma, irritable bowel spasm.

Home Remedies for backache #14: Wild Yam**—Dioscorea villosa

• Indicated for backache characterized by sharp, knife-like sensations.

• A relaxant used for pain originating in the digestive system, gall bladder, nervous system, uterus. Supplies precursors for adrenal cortisol.

Home Remedies for Arteriosclerosis

Arteriosclerosis or hardening of the arteries is the leading cause of disease and death in America, causing heart disease, stroke, kidney disease and problems with circulation in the limbs.

Arteriosclerosis occurs due to oxidative damage to the lining of the arteries, infiltration with fat-filled cells and formation of plaques and clots.

Risk factors include smoking, blood sugar disorders, obesity, an excess of "bad" cholesterol or LDL and high homocysteine levels, as well as a diet high in refined carbohydrates and trans fatty acids (i.e. processed oils). Damage to the arterial wall may also be due to chronic viral or bacterial infection.

Supplementation with folic acid, B12 and B6, CoO10, selenium, omega 3 oils and antioxidants would cut the risk of Arteriosclerosis and heart disease to a fraction of its current rate.

Herbal treatment for hardening of the arteries relies upon the strong antioxidant power of many plants, preventing the arterial damage that acts as a site for the development of plaque. They also prevent oxidation of LDL cholesterol, which leads to arterial deposits.

Some herbs can remove existing arteriosclerosis, returning elasticity to arteries. Such plants have multiple benefits, such as toning the heart, reducing cholesterol and preventing blood cell clumping and clot formation. The central herb for the heart is hawthorn, while a combination or rotating schedule of several other healing plants will maximize their long-term benefit.

Home remedies for Arteriosclerosis

Home remedies for Arteriosclerosis #1: Arjuna**—Terminalia arjuna

• Main Ayurvedic heart tonic, normalizes the heart's rhythm, improves blood flow in coronary arteries. Reduces cholesterol; antibacterial.

• Improves symptoms of congestive heart failure and reduces angina pain.

Home remedies for Arteriosclerosis #2: Bromelain**—Pineapple/Ananas comosus

- A proteolytic enzyme derived from the stem of the pineapple plant.

- Reduces blood platelet "stickiness" and subsequent clot formation.

- Decreases the inflammatory response to artery injury or irritation.

Home remedies for Arteriosclerosis #3: Cayenne**—Capsicum frutescens

- Stimulates blood flow, lowers cholesterol; may affect arteriosclerosis.

- Reduces risk of blood clotting, increases heart output.

- Increases capillary resistance, strengthens blood vessels in the limbs.

- Improves peripheral circulation and warms the hands and feet.

Home remedies for Arteriosclerosis #4: Curcamin***—Turmeric/Curcuma longa

- Antioxidant power eight times more potent than Vitamin E; prevents damage to blood vessel walls to prevent onset of arteriosclerosis.

- Improves blood flow in arteries, while strengthening blood vessels.

- Significantly reduces cholesterol, serum lipids, blood clot formation.

Home remedies for Arteriosclerosis #5: Garlic ***—Allium sativa

- In one two-year study, reduced the size of arterial plaque by 20%.

- Blocks the formation of new plaque.

- Lowers cholesterol and triglycerides (by 10-20%), lowers LDL and raises HDL cholesterol; prevents oxidation and thus damage to arteries.

- A natural anti-coagulant; helps dissolve potential clots (fibrinolysis).

Home remedies for Arteriosclerosis #6: Ginger* *—Zingiber officinale

- Thins the blood, decreases platelet aggregation and lowers cholesterol.

- Decreases blood pressure and reduces hardening of the arteries.

- Antioxidant, contains potent proteolytic enzymes; prevents clots.

Home remedies for Arteriosclerosis #7: Ginkgo***—Ginkgo biloba

- Increases microcirculation to all parts of the body, heart, limbs, brain.

- Blood-thinning activity, inhibits clot formation and inflammation.

- Antioxidant; strengthens, tones arteries, improving their elasticity.

Home remedies for Arteriosclerosis #8: Grape Seed Extract***—Vitis vinifera

- Antioxidant power 20 times that of vitamin C, 50 times vitamin E.

- Prevents arteriosclerosis and improves circulation in arteries, veins.

- Lowers cholesterol and actually shrinks existing deposits in arteries.

- Reduces blood cell agglutination, preventing clots, heart attack, stroke.

- Proanthocyanidins (OPCs) strengthen vessel walls, capillaries.

Home remedies for Arteriosclerosis #9: Guggul***—Commiphora gulgul

• Prevents arteriosclerosis, while reducing existing plaque in arteries.

• Lowers cholesterol and triglycerides as well as medical drugs. Lowers total cholesterol up to 30% in 3 months, raising HDL and lowering LDL.

Home remedies for Arteriosclerosis #10: Hawthorn***—Crataegus oxycantha

Traditionally used over a long term to remove arteriosclerotic deposits.

• Essential cardiotonic that strengthens the heart muscle (myocardium).

• Prevents cardiovascular disease by dilating the coronary vessels.

• Improves blood and oxygen to the heart, coronary arteries and tissues.

• Strengthens contraction of the heart muscles, regulates blood pressure.

Home remedies for Arteriosclerosis #11: Shlitake**—Lentinus edodes

• Protective antioxidant, inhibits the formation of arteriosclerotic plaque.

• Helps prevent cardiovascular disease, stroke and diabetes.

• Lowers cholesterol up to 15%, prevents clots, regulates blood sugar.

Home Remedies for Bladder Infection

The term UTI includes bladder irritation, as well as infection caused by various microorganisms.

Bladder infection conditions occur more often in women, due to anatomical differences.

In middle-aged men, however, a swollen prostate is the typical cause for urinary retention and infection. Underlying causes include nutritional deficiencies and immune susceptibility, as well as the more obvious irritations from intercourse, tight clothing, spices, coffee, tea, medicines, alcohol or high sugar in the urine. Food allergies may be a significant factor, especially in children.

Herbs for the urinary tract infection generally have diuretic effects, to flush out infection and inflammation by-products. Many are also antimicrobial, either destroying microorganisms or stimulating the body to do so. Along with quelling inflammation, other plants help heal irritated mucus membrane linings of the bladder, urethra and ureter, and the kidney tubules.

In most cases, simple bladder infection can be easily and effectively dealt with using the herbs below. In cases where antibiotic resistant bacteria are involved, or where no bacteria are detected, as in interstitial cystitis, herbs become even more important and uniquely effective.

Home remedies for bladder Infection

Home remedies for bladder Infection #1: Buchu**—Agathosma or Barosma betulina

• A diuretic and urinary antiseptic for cystitis, urethritis, prostatitis.

• Tones the urinary tract and helps prevent stones; treats bedwetting.

• Helpful for prostate enlargement and resulting bladder infections.

Home remedies for bladder Infection #2: Corn Silk**—Zea mays

• A soothing diuretic for irritation of the bladder, urethra and prostate.

• Relieves urinary tract inflammation and bedwetting in children.

• Effective for difficult and scant urination, cystitis and kidney stones.

Home remedies for bladder Infection #2: Couchgrass*—Agropyron repens

• A soothing urinary demulcent, useful for infection or inflammation of the prostate, urethra or bladder. Useful in kidney stone and gravel.

Home remedies for bladder Infection #3: Cranberry***—Vacciniurn macrocarpon

• Reduces bacteria and prevents them from adhering to the bladder walls.

• Can be taken as a preventive in people with recurring infections.

• Safe and effective during pregnancy, for children and the elderly.

• Mildly acidifies the urine, eliminating alkaline bacteria, (i.e. E. coli).

• Reduces effectiveness of uva ursi; should not be used together.

Home remedies for bladder Infection #4: Goldenrod**—Solidago virgaurea

Diuretic, anti-inflammatory and antiseptic effects for cystitis, urethritis.

Pain-relieving and antifungal, tones the bladder, soothes irritation. Safe and mild action; does not deplete body's electrolytes/potassium.

Home remedies for bladder Infection #5: Goldenseal***—Hydrastis canadensis

Anti-inflammatory and antimicrobial; destroys many types of bacteria.

• Especially effective for chronic cystitis or stubborn urinary mucus.

• Healing effect on bladder linings, stops bleeding, heals ulcerations.

Home remedies for bladder Infection #6: Gravel Root—Joe Pye
Weed/Eupatorium

Home remedies for bladder Infection #7: Horsetail**—Equisetum arvense

Acute urinary tract infection; safe during pregnancy or weakened states.

Diuretic effects, but does not deplete the body of salts or electrolytes.

Home remedies for bladder Infection #8: Juniper Berry*—Juniperus communis

A powerful diuretic, antispasmodic and strong antibiotic for cystitis.

▪ Must not be used for prolonged periods or in kidney infections.

Home remedies for bladder Infection #9: Marshmallow***—Althea officinalis

A soothing demulcent to the lining of the urinary tract.

Use for acute inflammation, typical of bladder infections.

Decreases inflammation in the respiratory, digestive or urinary tract.

Home remedies for bladder Infection #10: Parsley Root*—Petroselinum crispum
Diuretic effects for cystitis, kidney stones. Soothes burning, itching, crawling in
the urethra. Avoid in kidney disease or pregnancy.

Helps symptoms of pain, frequent desire, urging, mucus discharges.

Home remedies for bladder Infection #11: Sarsaparilla***—Smilax officinalis

For cystitis, kidney infections, bladder stones, kidney colic, bedwetting. " A blood

purifier that is antiseptic, anti-inflammatory; controls itching.

Diuretic. Rheumatic or skin problems (psoriasis) with urinary irritation.

Home remedies for bladder Infection #12: Uva ursi***—Arctostaphylos uva ursi

Urinary disinfectant and antiseptic, effective for many types of bacteria. "
Diuretic and astringent for chronic and acute urinary problems. " Avoid acidic
foods—and cranberry—which decrease its effectiveness.

Home remedies for bladder Infection #13: Yarrow**—Achillea millefolium

Increases urination, has antimicrobial effects, stops bleeding. Anti-inflammatory
properties, while soothing bladder spasms. Tones the urinary tract and acts as a
mild pain reliever in infections.

Home Remedies Indigestion

NUTRITIONAL SUPPLEMENTS FOR INDIGESTION

Indigestion Home Remedies #1: Many people with acid reflux find their symptoms improve if they take supplements containing betaine hydrochloride (HC1). Apparently, if the level of acid in the stomach is too low, the sphincter muscle separating the stomach and the esophagus can loosen, allowing what acid there is to escape up into the esophagus. Betaine HC1 increases the acidity of the stomach and helps prevent this problem. It is available in a variety of formulas, both on its own and with additional digestive enzymes. Follow the dosage directions on the product label and take it immediately after meals.

Indigestion Home Remedies #2: If your main complaint occurs within thirty minutes of eating, take a full-spectrum digestive-enzyme supplement providing 5,000 international units of lipase, 2,500 international units of amylase, and 300 international units of protease, plus 500 to 1,000 milligrams of pancreatin, immediately after the two largest meals of the day to ensure complete digestion.

Note: Long-term supplementation with pancreatin is not advised, as it can cause your pancreas to reduce its own production of this important enzyme. Overuse also has the potential to cause nausea or diarrhea. After two months on pancreatin, discontinue use and monitor your reaction. If you find that your digestive problems recur, discuss pancreatin supplementation with your health-care provider.

Indigestion Home Remedies #3: Glutamine can help soothe irritation in the

gastrointestinal tract. Try taking 500 milligrams of L-glutamine two to three times daily for up to one month.

Indigestion Home Remedies #4: Take probiotic supplements of acidophilus and/or bifidobacteria. For indigestion, powdered or liquid formulas are the best choice; these work in the stomach, while capsules open in the intestines. Tablets are not usually as effective, and must be chewed thoroughly.

Indigestion Home Remedies #5: Acidophilus powder can be taken any time for indigestion—simply take 1/4 to 1/2 teaspoon as needed. If you must use capsules, open them and pour the contents onto your tongue rather than swallowing them whole. If you are allergic to milk, select a dairy-free formula.

Indigestion Home Remedies #6: Vitamin E soothes the stomach. Choose the mixedtocopherol or d-alpha tocopherol form, not dl-alpha-tocopherol. Begin by taking 200 international units daily and gradually increase the dosage until you are taking 400 international units once or twice daily.

Note: If you have high blood pressure, limit your intake of supplemental vitamin E to a total of 400 international units daily. If you are taking an anticoagulant (blood thinner), consult your physician before taking supplemental vitamin E.

HERBAL TREATMENT FOR INDIGESTION

Indigestion Home Remedies #7: Aloe vera juice helps to clear and resolve an upset stomach that feels "burning." Make sure to get a food- grade product. Take 1 tablespoon diluted in 6 ounces of water up to three times daily. Use it sparingly; it can be a strong cathartic.

Indigestion Home Remedies #8: Gentian root is a bitter herb that has been used for centuries throughout Europe to enhance digestion, especially of proteins and fats. Take 500 milligrams twice a day, with meals.

Indigestion Home Remedies #9: Ginger is a notable digestive aid. It aids digestion, enhances assimilation, and reduces nausea. Take one or two 500-milligram capsules as needed.

Indigestion Home Remedies #10: Deglycyrrhizinated licorice (DGL) can be amazingly helpful. Chew two 250- to 500-milligram lozenges with a glass of water twenty minutes before each meal.

Note: Ordinary licorice can elevate blood pressure, and should not be taken on a daily basis for more than five days in a row. DGL should not have this effect, however.

Indigestion Home Remedies #11: Peppermint is a time-tested, time-honored herb that is very effective for all forms of indigestion. It enhances digestion, speeds the emptying time of the stomach, and reduces flatulence. Drink peppermint tea with meals.

Note: If you are using peppermint tea and also taking a homeopathic preparation, allow one hour between the two. Otherwise, the strong smell of the mint may interfere with the action of the homeopathic remedy.

Home Remedies Abscess

An abscess is a local accumulation of pus. It can occur almost anywhere on or in the body, but it most frequently occurs on the skin and on the gums of the mouth.

Abscesses can be very tender and painful and are marked by inflammation, swelling, heat, redness, and often fever. Abscesses are caused by an infection, so orthodox medical doctors often treat them with antibiotics. But herbs are an effective and safe alternative, without the side effects of antibiotics.

Abscess Home Remedies #1:

SKIN-ABSCESS—FIGHTING TEA

3o drop echinacea tincture

6o drop.a yerba mania tincture

1 cup warm water

Combine all the ingredients. Take up to five times per day to stimulate the immune system and help eliminate the infection.

Abscess Home Remedies #2:

TOPICAL WASH FOR SKIN AND GUM ABSCESSES

1 to 2 teaspoons barberries

1 tablespoon white oak bark

1 teaspoon echinacea root

1 teaspoon granulated Oregon grape root

2 cups boiling water

Combine the herbs in a glass container. Pour the boiling water over the herbs and soak for 3 to 4 hours; strain. Use three times a day as a wash. If you are using this tea to treat a gum abscess, be sure to swish the liquid around in your mouth for several minutes before spitting it out.

DIETARY GUI IELINES FOR ABSCESS

Abscess Home Remedies #3: Drink at least ten 8-ounce glasses of pure water daily until the abscess heals.

Abscess Home Remedies #4: Eat plenty of steamed leafy green vegetables and sea vegetables to ensure a good supply of vitamins and minerals needed for healing.

Abscess Home Remedies #5: Eat fresh pineapple. Fresh pineapple contains bromelain, which is very effective at reducing inflammation.

Abscess Home Remedies #6: Eliminate from your diet all fried foods and anything containing refined sugar, which slow healing.

NUTRITIONAL SUPPLEMENTS FOR ABSCESS

Abscess Home Remedies #7: Blue-green algae contains many trace minerals that are needed for healing and that are missing in the average diet. Take 300 milligrams two or three times daily.

Abscess Home Remedies #8: Colloidal silver is a liquid mineral supplement that fights infection. Take 10 drops three to four times daily

Abscess Home Remedies #9: If you must take antibiotics, restore the body's "friendly" bacteria by taking a probiotic supplement, such as acidophilus and/or bifido bacteria, as recommended on the product label. If you are allergic to milk, select a dairy-free formula. Colostrum is another effective probiotic that can be taken on a rotating basis with acidophilus and bifidobacteria. Take 300 milligrams three times daily, between meals.

Abscess Home Remedies #10: Vitamin C and bioflavonoids improve the immune response and help to reduce inflammation. Take 1,000 milligrams of vitamin C three to five times daily and 500 milligrams of mixed bioflavonoids three to four times daily.

HERBAL TREATMENT

Abscess Home Remedies #11: Cat's claw enhances the immune response and has antibacterial properties. Take 500 milligrams of standardized extract three times a day until the abscess clears.

Note: Do not use cat's claw if you are pregnant or nursing, or if you are an organ-transplant recipient. Use it with caution if you are taking an anticoagulant (blood thinner).

Abscess Home Remedies #12: Echinacea and goldenseal have antibacterial properties and also boost the body's natural immune response. They are helpful for fighting virtually any type of infection. Take one dose of an echinacea and goldenseal combination formula supplying 250 to 500 milligrams of echinacea and 150 to 300 milligrams of goldenseal three to four times daily for up to one week.

Cramping Home Remedies

Cramping can occur in any hollow organ of the body, but here we are primarily dealing with spasms in the digestive tract. Causes are many, including indigestion, infection or inflammation anywhere in the intestinal tract. Infantile colic, due to weak digestion, food allergies and gas formation, is a trial for both mother and baby. In adults, a variety of irritants can cause acute cramps, while chronic gut toxicity causes cramps relating to dysbiosis, irritable bowel and colitis. In all cases, underlying causes need to be addressed while painful spasms are being alleviated.

Antispasmodic herbs can provide a simple and non-toxic approach to calming painful cramps and colic. Such herbs are often nervines as well, providing sedative and calming effects for jangled nerves.

Other needed herbs are also carminatives, helping expel excess gas, and digestive tonics with anti-inflammatory effects. Deeper problems can be improved with herbal detoxification programs for the intestines and liver. In colic, food allergies in the baby, or in a mother who is breastfeeding, need to be identified and eliminated, until the immune system can be re-regulated to eliminate these sensitivities. The same holds true for adults.

Cramping Home Remedies

Home remedies for cramp #1: Anise***—Pimpinella anisum

• An important infant and child remedy for colic and general cramping.

• Antispasmodic and carminative, eases nausea, indigestion, bloating.

• Safe, gentle, tasty; can work via the breast milk. Improves appetite.

Home remedies for cramp #2: Caraway**—Carum carvi

• Similar to fennel and anise, relieves intestinal colic or cramps associated with gas, bloating, digestive upset, nausea and indigestion.

• Gentle enough for children, also good for menstrual cramping.

Home remedies for cramp #3: Catnip***—Nepeta cataria

• Relieves intestinal spasm and gas, diarrhea; mild relaxing effect.

• Relieves upset stomach, indigestion. Safe in children and the elderly.

• Is especially effective for intestinal or gastric upset of a nervous origin.

• Gentle and calming; sedates anxiety, reduces fever, eases headaches.

Home remedies for cramp #4: Chamomile***—Matricaria recutita

• Effective antispasmodic and colic remedy, soothes indigestion; anti-inflammatory and antiseptic. Calms irritability, restlessness, insomnia.

• Antidotes effects on nursing child of coffee or drug use by mother.

Home remedies for cramp #5: Cramp Bark***—Viburnum opulus

• Stronger antispasmodic than black haw; relieves painful cramping in abdomen, stomach, uterus or bladder. Relieves back pain, neuralgia.

• Effective for menstrual cramps, false labor pains. Helps with leg cramps.

Home remedies for cramp #6: Dill***—Anethum graveolens

• Relieves intestinal spasms, cramps, infantile colic and indigestion.

• Dispels gas and calms and improves the digestion; antibacterial action.

• Increases breast milk, which carries antispasmodic effects to the infant.

Home remedies for cramp #7: Fennel**—Foeniculum vulgare

• Stimulates digestion, relieves colic, flatulence, bloating and distension.

• Like anise and caraway, also used in coughs, as an antispasmodic and expectorant.

Increases breast milk; has a reputation as a longevity herb.

Home remedies for cramp #8: Kava Kava**—Piper methysticum

• Muscle relaxant and antispasmodic for internal organs and muscle tension. Sedative pain and cramp reliever, reduces sensitivity to pain.

• Strongly reduces anxiety, relieves sleeplessness, is a mild antiseptic.

Home remedies for cramp #9: Lemon Balm* *—Melissa officinalis

• Eases cramps and spasms, gas and bloating, indigestion and colic pains, gastric

acidity. Useful for problems related to stress and anxiety.

• A good children's herb; soothes anxiety, irritability, restlessness.

Home remedies for cramp #10: Licorice**—Glycyrrhiza glabra

• Demulcent and anti-inflammatory, decreases the spasms of gastritis or
intestinal distress, relieves stomach ulcers and body's stress response.

• Mild laxative, assists in the body's clearing of poorly digested foods.

Home remedies for cramp #11: Peppermint**—Mentha piperta

• Digestive antispasmodic; relieves colic, spasm, spastic constipation.

• Carminative, dispels gas and distention, with pain-relieving action.

• Stomachic, improves digestion, stimulates secretions and bile output.

Home remedies for cramp #12: Valerian**—Valeriana officinalis

• A sedative and antispasmodic, relaxing intestinal cramps, muscle tension.
Relieves spasms and pain related to anxiety and emotional upset.

• For cramps with diarrhea, or after eating. Promotes restful sleep.

Home remedies for cramp #13: Wild Yam***—Dioscorea villosa

• Important antispasmodic for cramps in any hollow organ; intestines, stomach or gall bladder spasm. For colic that is relieved by stretching.

• Helps with gas and flatulence, belching, indigestion, upset from tea.

Home remedies for cramp #14: Yarrow*—Achillea millefolium

• A digestive antispasmodic, anti-inflammatory and pain reliever.

• For cramping pains or stomachache, distension, or gas pain.

• A sedative and tranquilizing herb that promotes tissue healing.

Homemade Remedies for Cough

A cough is a natural reaction, designed to expel irritating, toxic material and mucus accumulations in the bronchial tubes. However, as everyone knows, even repeated coughing is sometimes ineffective at ridding the body of these irritants, and itself become fatiguing and debilitating.

For coughs, there are herbs that have a specific affinity to the chest and lung area (pectorals).

Some herbs are true antitussives or cough-suppressants (coltsfoot, horehound, wild cherry bark, licorice) or are just effective antispasmodics. Many are demulcents, soothing irritated bronchial tubes while others are expectorants, helping expel tough, adherent mucus. The powerful antibacterial and antiviral properties of many of these same plants makes them an excellent choice for getting at both symptoms and causes.

Many herbal cough formulas are available that combine these various properties and are often superior to a single herb.

The herbs below represent the best of literally hundreds of herbal cough medicines.

Note that demulcent herbs are more applicable to dry coughs (licorice, slippery elm, mullein, althea), while astringent plants are more suitable to moist, rattly or congested coughs (anise, eyebright, cowslip, thyme, eucalyptus). See also Asthma Colds & Flu

Home Remedies for Cough #1:

Anise***—Pimpinella anisum

• Helps expel mucus, while being anti-inflammatory, antispasmodic.

• For colds, coughs, bronchitis; also reduces nausea, gas, bloating.

• Safe for infants and children; a popular colic and indigestion remedy.

• Often mixed with other herbs for above effects and sweet licorice taste.

Home Remedies for Cough #2: Coltsfoot**—Tussilago farfara

• Expels mucus, soothes irritated membranes and suppresses coughs.

• Coughs related to upper respiratory infections (colds), acute and chronic bronchitis, asthma, hoarseness, whooping cough and emphysema.

• See Dosage. Should not be used excessively or for prolonged periods.

Home Remedies for Cough #3: Cowslip**—Primula veris

• Strong antispasmodic and expectorant for rattly coughs, chronic bronchitis with thick white mucus. Warming and sedative effects.

Home Remedies for Cough #4: Elecampane***—Inula helenium

412

- For coughs and bronchitis, including chronic cough; gentle for children.

- Soothing expectorant; helps expel excess mucus, antibacterial effects.

- Relieves bronchial spasm in asthma, emphysema, bronchitis.

Home Remedies for Cough #5: Eucalyptus**—Eucalyptus globulus

- Expectorant, natural decongestant, often used in rubs and liniments.

- Opens bronchial passages, clears mucus during colds, flu, bronchitis.

- Natural antiseptic. Use as an inhalant or lotion; high toxicity internally.

Home Remedies for Cough #6: Grindelia**—Gumweed/Grindelia camporum

- For coughs of bronchitis and asthma, whooping cough or viral coughs.

- Clears tough mucus, improves breathing and smothering tendency on falling asleep.

Slows rapid heartbeat and reduces high blood pressure.

Home Remedies for Cough #7: Horehound***—Marrubiurn vulgare

- Loosens mucus, soothes coughs; aids stuffy nose, sore throat and colds.

- For bronchitis, wheezing congested chest, with inability to expel mucus.

- Treats asthma or chronic lung conditions with poor expectoration.

Home Remedies for Cough #8: Hyssop* * *—Hyssopus officinalis

• Relieves coughs, bronchitis; loosens and expels mucus accumulations.

• Best in chronic coughs; a tonic, stimulating herb that speeds recovery.

• Asthmatic coughs in adults, children. Promotes sweat in colds and flu.

Home Remedies for Cough #9: Irish Moss*--Chondrus crispus

• A mucilaginous, jelly-like seaweed used in many respiratory conditions.

• A soothing demulcent used for irritating coughs, inflamed membranes.

• An expectorant for phlegm and mucus, encourages a productive cough.

Home Remedies for Cough #10: Licorice**—Glycyrrhiza glabra

• A powerful cough suppressant, soothing expectorant, demulcent and anti-inflammatory. Treats bronchitis, coughs, asthma, sore throats.

Home Remedies for Cough #11: Lomatium**—Lomatium dissectum

• Powerful antiviral, antibacterial herb, kills at least ten bacterial strains.

• Eliminates a broad range of acute and chronic viruses.

• For flus, cold, chronic bronchitis, viral pneumonia. Expels hard mucus.

Home Remedies for Cough #12: Lungwort* —Sticta pulmonaria

• For cough and bronchitis. For dry hacking night cough, preventing sleep.

• Treats lingering coughs after measles, flu, colds, whooping cough.

• Soothes tickling in throat, bronchi, where one cough incites another.

Home Remedies for Cough #13: Maidenhair Fern*—Adiantum cappillus

• Used for coughs, bronchitis, asthma and general respiratory disorders.

• Soothes sore throats, expels mucus, helps chronic sinus congestion.

Home Remedies for Cough #14: Mullein**—Verbascum thapsus

• Traditional cough remedy that soothes dry and inflamed throat and bronchi, clears

mucus, allays bronchial spasms, shrinks swollen glands.

• Useful in colds, flu, bronchitis, asthma and even emphysema.

Home Remedies for Spider Veins

As 75 percent of people over the age of sixty-five know, veins that have become swollen, raised, and snakelike are called Spider Veins. If one or more of the one-way valves in superficial veins no longer functions normally, the blood headed back to the heart can pool or even flow backward. This stretches the vein and makes it impossible for other nearby valves to close properly as well. The vein becomes swollen and kinked, and blood stagnates in the vein. The veins turn purple, dark blue, or cranberry in color.

Spider Veins are most common on the thighs, the backs of the calves, the insides of the legs, and the ankles. In addition to being cosmetically displeasing, Spider Veins often feel heavy, burn, itch, or throb, and the feet and ankles can swell.

The legs may feel hot and heavy and become sensitive to pressure. Symptoms generally worsen during the day, especially with prolonged standing.

The severity of the appearance of the Spider Veins does not necessarily correspond to the severity of the associated pain and soreness.

People with only a few visible varicosities can suffer from severe pain from them.

Spider Veins run in families, and affect women more frequently because of premenstrual or menopausal hormones, birth control pills, and pregnancy. In fact, they occur in 40 percent of pregnant women. Other factors that contribute to Spider Veins include advancing age, muscular atrophy in the legs, poor circulation, smoking, prolonged bed rest, overweight, lack of exercise, prolonged standing or sitting, tight clothing, high heels, excessive heavy lifting, and chronic constipation.

In addition to being painful and tiring, Spider Veins can cause other problems. These include blood clots and inflammation in the veins, and bleeding (either under the skin or on the surface) if the distended vein is accidentally cut or bumped.

The presence of many varicosities prevents the delivery of enough nutrients and oxygen to the tissues of the legs and delays removal of wastes from leg tissues. Then the skin around the varicosities may become very thin, discolored, hardened, and prone to ulcers.

Very tiny dilated capillaries, usually on the face, legs, and thighs, are called spider veins. They are typically a red or bluish color and can be short unconnected lines or come together in a "sunburst" pattern or a spiderweblike pattern just under the surface of the skin. They are not an early sign of Spider Veins and are not a dangerous problem.

Spider veins often run in families, and tend to be more common in women, especially with the hormonal changes of puberty and pregnancy.

Injury to a part of the body or wearing tight hosiery may bring out unwanted spider veins in the involved area. Spider veins also occur on the face in those with fair skin, rosacea, and chronic, unprotected sun exposure.

Home remedies for spider veins

Home remedies for spider veins #1: Horse-chestnut seed offers perhaps the best herbal relief for the swelling, pain, itching, fatigue, and tenseness associated with varicose and spider veins. Clinical studies show that horse chestnut improves circulation in the legs, decreases inflammation, and strengthens the capillaries and veins. Combine ten parts distilled witch hazel with one part tincture of horse chestnut and apply this mixture externally to the affected areas as needed to help ease discomfort. Look for an extract of horse chestnut that provides a daily dosage of 50 milligrams of aescin, one of the key compounds that strengthens capillary cells and reduces fluid leakage. You can also take 500 milligrams of oral horse chestnut three times a day. It usually takes about 3 months to see benefits, so be patient.

Caution: Do not exceed the recommended oral dosage of horse chestnut extract, because larger doses can be toxic.

Home remedies for spider veins #2:Bilberry extract stimulates new capillary formation, strengthens capillary walls, and enhances the effect of vitamin C in reducing blood-vessel fragility. Take 20 to 40 milligrams three times a day.

Home remedies for spider veins #3: Butcher's broom extract improves varicosities by constricting and strengthening veins. Take 300 milligrams three times a day.

Home remedies for spider veins #4: Gingko biloba extract enhances tissue oxygenation and circulation. Take 40 milligrams three times a day.

Home remedies for spider veins #5:Grapeseed extract also improves circulation. Take 50 milligrams three times a day.

Home remedies for spider veins #6: Gotu kola extract is helpful for venous insufficiency, water retention in the ankles, foot swelling, and varicose veins. Take 200 milligrams three times a day.

Home remedies for spider veins #7:Hawthorn extract contains vitamin C, bioflavonoids, zinc, and sulfur, all of which are helpful for varicose veins. Take 200 milligrams three times a day

Home remedies for spider veins #8: Distilled witch hazel is soothingly astringent when applied to areas with varicosities by means of a cotton ball dipped in the extract.

Several studies in animals have shown that witch hazel helps to strengthen blood vessels as well.

Supplements for Spider Veins

Vitamin C, bioflavonoids, and vitamin E help to improve circulation and reduce pain from varicosities. Bioflavonoids also strengthen venous walls and connective tissue that supports blood vessels, and vitamin E also acts as a blood thinner to improve circulation. Take 1,000 milligrams of vitamin C and 300 milligrams of a bioflavonoid complex three times daily, and 200 international units of vitamin E twice daily. Take an additional 1,000 milligrams of rutin daily.

Essential fatty acids also help to decrease pain from varicose veins. Take 500 to 1,000 milligrams of black currant seed, borage, or evening primrose oil a day to reduce pain.

Take 25,000 international units of beta-carotene daily.

Take a vitamin-B complex plus an additional 60 milligrams of vitamin B6 daily for several months.

Herbs and Skin Care.

From the Egyptian Queen Cleopatra to the Japanese geishas, all used herbs to protect and rejuvenate their skin, and until the end of the 19th century, for women, herbs were the most important part of the process of looking young and healthy. Their cosmetic tools were natural oils extracted carefully from plants that their mothers had used for the same purpose.

By the middle of the 20th century, the use of herbs was regarded as old fashioned, and we were told that the best products to use for the care of our skin were the ones made in a chemical laboratory. Petrochemicals were blossoming and big corporations started to bombard the public with clever advertising, making them believe that their new synthetic and chemical fill creams were the most effective way of skin care. That's how we forgot that plants were used for hundreds of years to treat skin disorders and to keep it beautiful and healthy.

Looking at the labels of some of these products manufactured by chemists makes me wonder who in their right mind would dare to open the container and spread the content on their faces. Some moisturizers and lotions contain Propylene, glycol, isopropyl and myristate as active ingredients, and that's not all, to get rid of the nasty smell of these chemicals. The manufacturer adds fragrances made from petroleum, the same substance that makes your car run.

You may be using a shampoo or cream that contains herbs and the label real "natural." Here is a tip, never believe the front label, believe what they are obligated by law to show on the label placed on the back of the container. All ingredients must be listed in a descending order, for example, if the front label reads "Primrose Shampoo" and the back label lists primrose near the bottom, then that product contains very little of the essential oil and chances are that chemicals like hexachlorophene, diazolidinyl and polyquarterium-10, nullify the effectiveness of any botanical substance they may contain. In addition, it has been shown that these chemicals produce

422

wrinkles, but don't worry they also sell creams for that too.

Many people are becoming wary of the adverse effects of chemically produced cosmetics, and you are one of them, that's why you are reading this book, you want to find an alternative. The idea of chemicals in your body is getting old and outdated and since they came to the market there has not been a change for the better. To the contrary, cosmetic surgeries are on the rise. If these products are so amazingly perfectly designed to protect and to prevent, why do we need so much cosmetic surgery?

Skin Care the Natural Way.

Our skin and hair can have different needs, that's why you should choose a preparation that matches your skin complexion and hair type. However, remember that your skin is a reflection of your general health, if you smoke, drink alcohol, or if you have hormonal fluctuations, poor diet, and don't exercise, chances are that your skin will show signs of damage that normal skin treatment will not repair.

To maintain a radiant complexion and healthy hair, eat a balance diet, reduce stress, also rest and relax as much as possible, exercise and use the herb preparations we recommend. All this will ensure that a sufficient blood supply is reaching the layers of the skin, which provides nutrients and oxygen needed to repair and generate new healthy skin tissue.

Herbs can provide all you need to care for your skin. In the next section you'll find some examples of the different properties of herbs and the way to use them.

DRY SKIN PREPARATIONS.

TIP:Did you know that yogurt, placed on the face helps bring water from the deeper layers of the skin to the surface, thus moisturizing your skin for the rest of the day?

Cleanser for Dry Skin.

2 ounces aloe vera gel.

1 tsp. Vegetable oil or jojoba oil or Saint John's Wort oil.

1 tsp. Glycerin.

½ tsp. Grapefruit seed extract.

8 drops Sandalwood essential oil.

4 drops rosemary essential oil.

Mix all ingredients and shake well before use. Apply with cotton balls and rinse with warm water.

Toner for Dry Skin.

Toners are used to improve the appearance of the skin, to soothe and to nourish. Men can use toners as aftershaves.

2 ounces aloe vera gel.

2 ounces orange-blossom water.

1 tsp. wine vinegar.

6 drops rose geranium essential oil.

4 drops sandalwood essential oil.

1 drop chamomile essential oil. *

800 UI vitamin E oil. (Puncture a gel capsule with a needle)

Mix all ingredients and shake well before use.

*The director of the Dermatologic Clinic at the University of Bonn, Germany found that chamomile cream gives a smooth, healthy appearance to rough, red skin faster than other creams and it also reduces the appearance of wrinkles.

Cream for Dry Skin.

3/4 ounces beeswax, shaved. (do not use paraffin)

1 cup vegetable oil.

1 cup of distilled water.

800 UI vitamin E (from a liquid gel)

24 drops rose geranium essential oil.

Heat beeswax and oil in a pot until beeswax melts (it should be warm enough to the touch but without discomfort). In a separate pot heat water until is warm to the touch. Remove the center part of your blender's lid and pour the water in. Turn the blender on high speed and slowly but steadily add the oil and wax mixture. The whole concoction should begin to solidify. Keep adding oil until the mixture does not take any more. Turn off the blender and using a spatula, place the cream in a wide mouthed container.

Facial Steam for Dry Skin.

3 cups of water.

1 drop rose geranium essential oil.

1 drop rosemary essential oil.

1 drop fennel essential oil.

1 drop peppermint essential oil.

Boil water, turn off heat and add essential oils. Place a towel over your head and over the pot, close your eyes and let the steam warm your face. After 15 minutes splash your face with cool water.

Facial Scrub for Dry Skin.

2 tbsp. Oatmeal.

1 tbsp. Cornmeal.

1 tsp. chamomile flowers.

1 tsp. lavender flowers.

1 tsp. elder flowers.

6 drops lavender essential oil.

Grind all dry ingredients in an electric coffee grinder, add essential oil and mix thoroughly. To use, place a small amount of the mixture on the palm of your hand and moisten with a few drops of water to create a paste, wet your face and apply scrub gently. Rinse with warm water.

OILY SKIN PREPARATIONS.

TIP:Did you know that strawberries ans strawberry leaves reduce the production of oil? Other herbs that have a similar effect are basil, eucalyptus, cedarwood, sage, lemon, and ylang-ylang.

Cleanser for Oily Skin.

2 ounces witch hazel.

1 tsp. vinegar.

1 tsp. glycerin.

½ tsp. grapefruit seed extract.

6 drops lemon essential oil.

2 drops cypress essential oil.

Mix all ingredients and shake well before use. Apply with cotton balls and rinse with warm water.

Facial Steam for Oily Skin.

3 cups of water.

1 drop of chamomile essential oil.

1 drop of lemongrass essential oil.

1 drop of lavender essential oil.

1 drop of rosemary essential oil.

Boil water, turn off heat and add essential oils. Place a towel over your head and over the pot, close your eyes and let the steam warm your face. After 15 minutes splash your face with cool water.

Toner for Oily Skin.

2 ounces witch hazel.

1 tbsp. aloe vera gel.

5 drops cedarwood essential oil.

3 drops lemon essential oil.

1 drop ylang-ylang essential oil.

Mix ingredients. Shake well before using.

MATURE SKIN TREATMENTS

The question is, why does skin wrinkle? As you grow older, your body produces fewer of the hormones that keep skin healthy and supplies less oil, protein and natural moisturizing factors which attract and hold water in the skin. This process tends to make the skin drier. As time goes by, collagen and elastin (fibers arranged in a mesh-like pattern) eventually lose their strength, leaving the skin without underlying support and causing it to wrinkle and sag.

Any person over 25 years of age has mature skin, lines start to form around age 30, if you smoke or spend too much time in the sun your skin will look older. Since mature skin does not produce as much oil and natural moisturizers, you will need to follow many of the treatments for dry skin. Herbs can be very important contributors to the development of new cells and several herbs like lavender, neroli, rosemary, rose, and fennel, have been nicknamed centuries ago "anti-aging herbs".

Antioxidants are also very important. They prevent the production of free radicals. These free radicals play an important role in all aspects of aging including hardening of the arteries. They are unstable, quickly multiplying molecules, which are increased by cigarette smoking and other pollutants. Many herbs and vitamins have antioxidant properties and are very powerful in stopping free radicals on their tracks. Some antioxidant herbs are gingko, witch hazel, and essential oil of rosemary, marjoram, and lavender.

Age Spot Remover.

1 tsp. grated horseradish root.

½ tsp. lemon juice.

½ tsp. vinegar.

3 drops rosemary essential oil.

Mix ingredients. Keep away from eyes. Apply as needed on affected areas.

Toner for Mature Skin.

2 ounces aloe vera gel.

2 ounces orange blossom water.

1 tsp. vinegar.

6 drops rose geranium essential oil.

4 drops frankincense essential oil.

4 drops carrot seed essential oil.

800 IU vitamin E oil.

Mix ingredients, apply as needed.

Blemish Remover.

1/4 cup of water.

1 tsp. Epson salts.

4 drops lavender essential oil.

Small cloth.

Mix water and salts, once the salts has dissolved, add lavender. Soak a cotton cloth and compress on affected area. When cloth cools soak it again and repeat several times.

HOME REMEDIES FOR CELLULITE

Cellulite is a type of female skin disorder that appears on thighs and bottom when you grow up which is the curse of many a woman's existence. There are many methods to remove cellulite but homemade remedies can also decrease cellulite. There are 10 great home remedies cellulite below, check them out!

Cellulite is one of the most common conditions found in women in the specific regions such as thighs,below the legs,pelvic region etc and by a statistics it is noticed that more than 90% of women are suffering from this problem and are very eager to know the treatment for this problem and to get rid from this problem. home remedies cellulite

Cellulite are fat deposits in the connective tissues that force themselves out when trapped. They would then push upwards underneath the skin causing those ugly bumps and lumps. Due to its appearance, cellulite is also referred to as cottage cheese skin, orange peel syndrome, and the mattress phenomenon. To be more specific, the connective tissues appear in a criss-cross pattern in males and in a vertical, mattress springs-like pattern in women.

Cellulite can be caused by a variety of factors such as hormonal factors, genetics, excess body fat, excessive dieting, changes in metabolism, stress, alteration of the connective tissue structure, micro-circulation impairment, and so on. The exact cause of cellulite, however, is not well understood as yet.

Cellulite treatments can be quite costly; it's a good thing that there are now ways to get rid of cellulite at home. More often than not, cellulite develops in areas like the abdomen, thighs, buttocks, that is, areas containing deep layers of fat for reserve. However, it can develop in other areas like breasts and upper arms, too. Furthermore, it appears worse during old age as the skin tends to become thinner with increasing age.

HOME REMEDIES CELLULITE

Home Remedies Cellulite #1: Frequent massages improve the body's lymphatic flow preventing future cellulite formation. This type of home remedy can be fun and beneficial to you too. Massaging the skin with a mixture of essential oils like rosemary, almond and sunflower can loosen that cellulite and eventually break them down.

Brushing and massaging the skin with a soft brush can help improve circulation, boost lymph drainage, and hence, heal cellulite. You can do a dry brushing before taking your shower, about three times in a week. Apart from improving cellulite, dry brushing shall also slough off dry skin and open up the pores. Consider using a medium-stiff shower brush for this purpose. It is suggested to use gentle, upward (towards the heart), circular movements rather than harsh strokes as they can break the blood vessels. See Remedy number 7 below.

Home Remedies Cellulite #2: Increasing intake of fruits and vegetable can improve your circulation, reduce cellulite formation and reduce your body weight. Berries, bananas, oats and bran, asparagus, and oranges are just some of the fruits that effectively bust cellulite. Mix them as often as you can in your daily diet and soon your cellulite will be reduced.

Home Remedies Cellulite #3: Massaging with oil containing almond oil, and rosemary oil is very effective in cellulite treatment. Mix each oil in equal ratio (1:1) and apply on the cellulite area like hips, buttocks, thighs.

Home Remedies Cellulite #4: Do physical exercises that target mostly on your thighs, stomach, buttocks, and hip areas.Engage in physical activity and exercise regularly, try running, cycling, etc. or opt for intense cardio workouts.

Home Remedies Cellulite #5: Avoid excess salt in your diet as it harms your body and increases the water level in your body.

Home Remedies Cellulite #6: One of the common home remedies for cellulite is coconut oil. Coconut oil massage is very effective in treating cellulite problems.

Home Remedies Cellulite #7: Take one-fourth of coconut oil into a glass jar. Add a mixture 6 drops of each cypress essential oil and geranium essential oil to the jar. Shake the jar well. Let the mixture rest for a few hours. Add two drops each of lemon oil and grapefruit oil to the mixture. Shake the resulting mixture vigorously. Keep in a cool dark place such as cupboard.

Massage the affected are gently for 10 minutes a day. Massaging boosts the circulatory and lymphatic system. Thus, you can try a cellulite reduction massage by way of finger kneading and hand kneading. Besides, you can go for the knuckle massage with your fists to help break up the fat deposits. Make sure you end the massage with heavy strokes moving upwards.

Home Remedies Cellulite #8: Ginkgo Biloba is a wonderful medicinal herb that improves blood circulation, stimulates the metabolism, and burns fat. Hence, it aids in natural treatment for cellulite. So, you can take dried ginkgo biloba extract. Herbs like sweet clover and Indian chestnut are also considered beneficial in this regard.

Home Remedies Cellulite #9: Cut down on toxins in your diet that come from smoking and intake of caffeinated and alcoholic beverages & highly processed foods that come in packages.

Home Remedies Cellulite #10: Limit your consumption of sugar and salt; they promote fluid retention.

Table of Content

"To my beloved Bianca, without your cooperation this couldn´t be possible"

CSRS